MEDITTERRANEAN DIET FOR ALZHEIMERS DISEASE AFTER 50

(Exercise Program Incorporated)

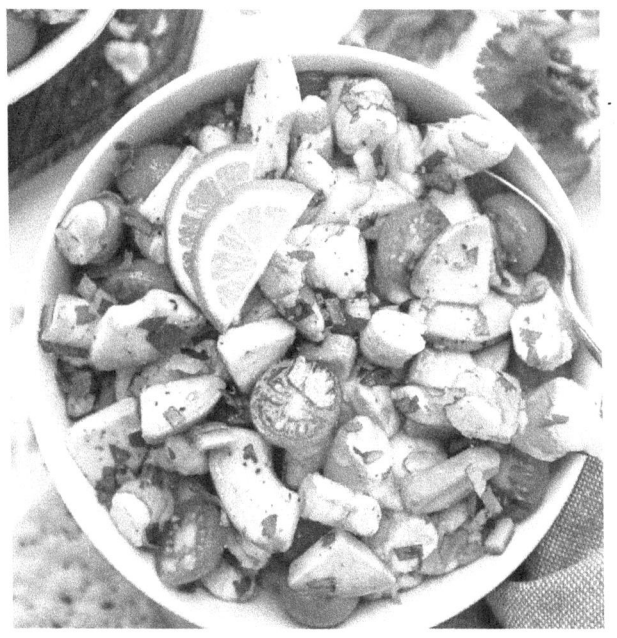

The Complete Tasty Nutritious Food and Lifestyle Guide to Preventing Cognitive Decline

EPIPHANY HUB PRINTS

MEDITTERRANEAN DIET FOR ALZHEIMERS DISEASE

Copyright © [2024] by [EPIPHANY HUB PRINTS]

All rights reserved. No part of this publication may be reproduced, distributed, or transmitted in any form or by any means, including photocopying, recording, or other electronic or mechanical methods, without the prior written permission of the publisher, except in the case of brief quotations embodied in critical reviews and certain other noncommercial uses permitted by copyright law.

TABLE OF CONTENTS

INTRODUCTION 9
CHAPTER 1: ALZHEIMER'S DISEASE 11
    Understanding Alzheimer's Disease 11
    The Role of Diet in Alzheimer's Disease: 12
    Key Components of the Mediterranean Diet and Their Potential Benefits for Alzheimer's Disease: 13
    Causes and Risk Factors 14
    Risk Factors for Alzheimer's Disease: 16
    Symptoms and Progression of Alzheimer's Disease: 19
    Alzheimer's Disease and the Mediterranean Diet: 21
CHAPTER 2: 23
OVERVIEW OF THE MEDITERRANEAN DIET 23
    Origins and History 23
    Essential Components of a Mediterranean Diet: 23
    Historical Context and Cultural Significance: 24
    Empirical Research and Alzheimer's Disease: 24
    Mechanisms of Action: 24
    Future Directions and Clinical Implications: 25
    Core Principles and Components 26
    Implications for Alzheimer's Disease Management: 27
    Health Benefits Beyond Nutrition 28
    The Mediterranean Diet: More Than Just Food: 28
    Scientific Proof of Its Effectiveness 31
CHAPTER 3: 34
NUTRITIONAL FOUNDATIONS OF THE MEDITERRANEAN DIET 34
    Emphasis on Plant-Based Foods 34
    The Role of Olive Oil: 34
    Nuts, Legumes, and Whole Grains: 35

Fish and Poultry: 35
Role of Healthy Fats and Oils: 36
Moderate Consumption of Fish and Poultry 38
Moderation is Key: 39
Limited Red Meat and Processed Foods 40
Processed Foods and Cognitive Health: 40
Practical Recommendations: 41
Whole Grains for Brain Health: 42
CHAPTER 4: MEDITERRANEAN DIET AND BRAIN HEALTH 44
Mechanisms Behind Diet-Brain Connection 44
Clinical Guidance and Future Directions: 45
Research on Mediterranean Diet and Brain Health 46
Mechanisms of Action: 47
Potential Benefits for Alzheimer's Disease Prevention and Management 48
Rich in Nutrients Components: 49
Anti-inflammatory Properties: 49
Blood Sugar Regulation: 50
Regulation of Gut Microbiota: 50
Social and Lifestyle Factors: 50
CHAPTER 5: 52
ANTI-INFLAMMATORY PROPERTIES OF THE MEDITERRANEAN DIET 52
Impact of Diet on Inflammatory Processes 52
Key Dietary Factors and Their Impact on Alzheimer's-Related Inflammation: 53
Practical Dietary Recommendations for Alzheimer's Prevention and Management: .. 54
Foods Rich in Anti-inflammatory Compounds 55
How Mediterranean Diet May Help Reduce Inflammation 57
CHAPTER 6: ANTIOXIDANTS AND NEUROPROTECTION 59
Oxidative Stress and Neurodegeneration. 59
The Part Oxidative Stress Plays in Alzheimer's Disability 59

Consequences of Oxidative Stress in Alzheimer's Disease 60

Therapeutic Strategies Targeting Oxidative Stress 61

Mediterranean-Style Dietary Supplements 61

Key Antioxidant-Rich Components of the Mediterranean Diet: 62

Understanding of Alzheimer's Pathophysiology 63

Potential Neuroprotective Mechanisms: 64

Round Anti-inflammatory Agents: 64

Emerging Neuroprotective Compounds and Therapies: 65

Lifestyle Interventions for Neuroprotection: 65

Challenges and Future Directions: 66

Incorporating Antioxidant-Rich Foods into Daily Diet 66

Types of Antioxidants: 67

Incorporating Antioxidant-Rich Foods into Your Daily Diet: 67

CHAPTER 7: GUT MICROBIOTA AND COGNITIVE HEALTH 70

Gut Microbiota and Alzheimer's Disease: 70

Influence of Diet on Gut Microbiota Composition: 70

Dietary Interventions for Alzheimer's Prevention and Management: 71

Future Directions and Clinical Implications: 72

Diversity of Gut Microbiota and the Mediterranean Diet 73

The Role of the Mediterranean Diet in Gut Microbiota Diversity: 74

Implications for Alzheimer's Disease Prevention: 74

CHAPTER 8: MEAL PLANNING AND RECIPES 78

Practical Tips for Adopting Mediterranean Diet 78

Sample Meal Plans for Different Dietary Preferences 81

CHAPTER 9: LIFESTYLE FACTORS AND ALZHEIMER'S PREVENTION 87

Beyond Diet: Importance of Physical Activity 87

I Am Even Little Adjustments Can Have an Impact: 88

Stress Management and Adequate Sleep 89

The Role of Sleep in Brain Health: 90

- Promoting Healthy Sleep Habits: 90
- Social Engagement and Mental Stimulation 91
- Strategies for Enhancing Social Engagement: 92
- The Importance of Mental Stimulation: 93
- Strategies for Promoting Mental Stimulation: 94

CHAPTER 10: 95

IMPLEMENTING THE MEDITERRANEAN DIET FOR ALZHEIMER'S PREVENTION 95

- Steps to Start Incorporating Mediterranean Diet 95
- Overcoming Challenges and Barriers 98
- Monitoring Progress and Adjusting Diet Accordingly 101
- Key Dietary Strategies: 101
- Practical Tips for Caregivers: 104

SEVEN (7) DAY MEDITERRENEAN MEAL PLAN FOR ALZHEIMERS DISEASE 106

- Day 1: 106
- Day 2: 106
- Day 3: 107
- Day 4: 107
- Day 5: 107
- Day 6: 108
- Day 7: 108

CONCLUSION 110

BONUS 112

EXERCISE PROGRAM FOR ALZHEIMERS DISEASE 112

- EXERCISE FOR YOUR BRAIN 112

INTRODUCTION

Despite the confusing array of modern nutrition fads, one nutritional approach—the Mediterranean diet—has endured the test of time, surviving across generations and cultural divides because of its enormous impact on health and welfare.

But its significance goes beyond only flavor; it provides a glimmer of hope amidst the gloom of neurodegenerative diseases like Alzheimer's. This is the place to start a novel exploration of the intersection between neuroscience and food: the "Mediterranean Diet for Alzheimer's Disease."

In this meticulously crafted book, we will explore the revolutionary potential of the Mediterranean diet in avoiding Alzheimer's disease. Through the use of a wealth of scientific data and culinary knowledge, we interpret the intricate connections between diet and mental health. We find that eating habits outside of the conventional medical environment have a major influence on cognitive performance.

Prepare to discover the vibrant mosaic of tastes, vibrant colors, and unparalleled nutritional value found in Mediterranean cuisine. Every dish, whether it originates from the rugged hills of Italy or the sun-kissed beaches of Greece, pays homage to ancient traditions entwined with the latest findings in nutritional science. But this is more than just a recipe book; it's a manual for reviving the mind and fueling the body to support the mind.

Through an exploration of these pages, we will be guided by the knowledge of both ancient civilizations and modern science to optimize the benefits of a Mediterranean diet for Alzheimer's prevention and management.

Equipped with knowledge, driven by preferences, and brimming with optimism for an improved tomorrow, let's go on this transformative journey in unison. Together, we can make Alzheimer's a disease that can be defeated by indulging in delicious, nutritious food instead of a fatal diagnosis.

CHAPTER 1: ALZHEIMER'S DISEASE

Understanding Alzheimer's Disease

The neurological condition known as Alzheimer's disease primarily affects the elderly. Memory, cognitive function, and ultimately the ability to do daily tasks steadily degrade as a result. Despite the lack of a proven cure for Alzheimer's disease, studies are still being conducted to see if some aspects of lifestyle, like diet, can help prevent or manage the illness.

The Mediterranean diet has garnered the greatest attention among these dietary approaches because of its potential neuroprotective properties and ability to impede the progression of Alzheimer's disease. In this article, we explore the nuances of Alzheimer's disease and how a Mediterranean diet could offer promising approaches to both prevention and treatment.

Understanding Alzheimer's Disease:

Alzheimer's disease is characterized by the accumulation of abnormal protein deposits in the brain, including tau tangles and beta-amyloid plaques. These pathogenic abnormalities result in neurons gradually degenerating and interfering with brain connectivity, which causes cognitive decline and memory loss. Though its exact origins are still unknown, a variety of factors, including genetics, lifestyle choices, and environmental factors, are likely to contribute to Alzheimer's disease.

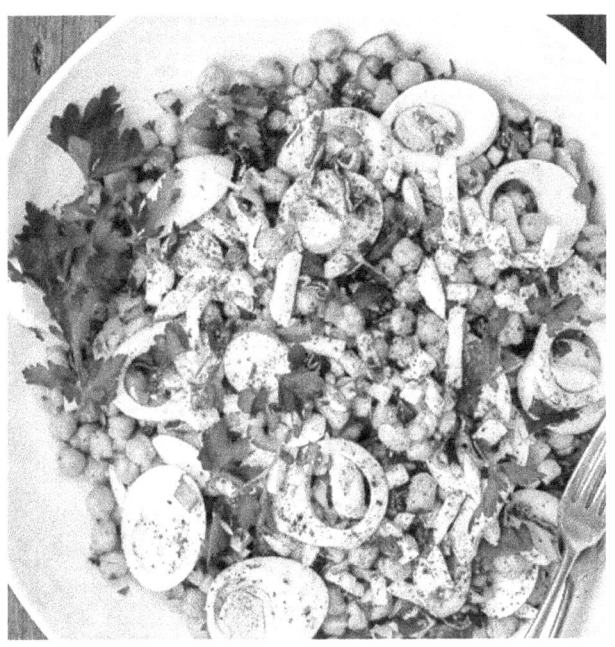

The Role of Diet in Alzheimer's Disease:

According to recent studies, diet plays a significant role in determining an individual's chance of developing Alzheimer's disease as well as how quickly it advances. Antioxidants, anti-inflammatory drugs, and omega-3 fatty acid-rich diets have been associated with a decreased incidence of dementia and cognitive decline. However, diets consisting in processed foods, sugar, and saturated fats have been linked to an increased risk of Alzheimer's disease.

A Nutritional Strategy for Preventing Alzheimer's Disease Is the Mediterranean Diet.

The historic eating habits of nations bordering the Mediterranean Sea, such Greece, Italy, and Spain, are the foundation of the Mediterranean diet. An abundance of fruits, vegetables, whole grains, legumes, nuts, seeds, and olive oil are some of its unique characteristics. eating dairy products, fish, and poultry in moderation.

Key Components of the Mediterranean Diet and Their Potential Benefits for Alzheimer's Disease:

Olive Oil: Rich in monounsaturated fats and polyphenols, olive oil contains anti-inflammatory and antioxidant

properties that may halt the formation of beta-amyloid plaques in the brain and prevent cognitive decline.
Fruits and Vegetables: Packed with vitamins, minerals, and phytochemicals, these foods promote brain repair and regeneration while reducing oxidative stress and inflammation.

Fish: Fish Fatty fish, such as mackerel, sardines, and salmon, are high in omega-3 fatty acids, which have been associated with a lower incidence of dementia and cognitive impairment.

Nuts and Seeds: Rich in antioxidants, fiber, and good fats, nuts and seeds improve cognitive function, boost brain health, and may even aid to maintain memory and learning capacity.

Whole Grains: Whole grains provide a steady stream of energy to the brain and are rich in nutrients, such as vitamin E, which has been linked to a decreased risk of Alzheimer's disease.

Clinical Support Supporting the Beneficial Effects of the Mediterranean Diet on Reducing the Risk of Alzheimer's Disease:

The Mediterranean diet has been shown to have protective effects on cognitive performance in a variety of observational studies and clinical trials. These studies show that a Mediterranean diet is associated with improved overall brain health, a slower pace of cognitive decline, and a lower risk of Alzheimer's disease.

Alzheimer's sufferers, their family, and the general public encounter a number of challenges. While there are currently no effective treatments for Alzheimer's disease, adopting a healthy lifestyle and making dietary adjustments may help reduce the risk of dementia and cognitive decline.

The Mediterranean diet, with its emphasis on whole foods, plant-based components, and healthy fats, offers a practical and long-term approach to improving brain function and potentially reducing the effects of Alzheimer's disease. By incorporating the Mediterranean diet's tenets into their regular eating routine, people may eventually protect their cognitive function and enhance their overall well-being in addition to their physical health.

Causes and Risk Factors

Among these diets, the Mediterranean diet is noteworthy because it may lower the risk of Alzheimer's forming and worsening. In this comprehensive guide, we will look at the origins and risk factors of Alzheimer's disease as well as how a Mediterranean diet may help manage and prevent the illness.

Alzheimer's Disease Causes Include:

Alzheimer's disease is caused by a complex interplay of behavioral, environmental, and hereditary factors. While the exact reason remains unknown, several significant mechanisms have been identified:

Beta-Amyloid Plaque Formation: When beta-amyloid protein fragments accumulate in the brain, plaques that obstruct nerve cell communication and worsen cognitive impairment develop.

Tau Protein Tangles: When tau protein, which is important for preserving the structural integrity of brain cells, is deviated from its usual range, tangles form inside neurons, which impede cell function and ultimately lead to cell death.

Neuro-inflammation: Prolonged inflammation in the brain is thought to cause damage to neurons and accelerate cognitive decline, both of which are important factors in the onset of Alzheimer's disease.

Oxidative Stress: When antioxidants and free radicals are not balanced, oxidative stress occurs. This damages cells and increases a person's risk of developing neurological conditions like Alzheimer's.

Genetic Factors: Although the majority of cases of Alzheimer's disease are sporadic, mutations in the APOE gene, for example, increase the risk of the illness developing.

Risk Factors for Alzheimer's Disease:

Several factors have been identified as increasing an individual's likelihood of developing Alzheimer's disease:

Age: The biggest risk factor for Alzheimer's is becoming older, with people over 65 accounting for the majority of cases.

Family History: If you have a first-degree relative with Alzheimer's disease, you may be genetically susceptible to the illness.

Cardiovascular Health: Individuals with high blood pressure, diabetes, obesity, and high cholesterol have an increased risk of Alzheimer's disease.

Sedentary Lifestyle: Lack of cognitive stimulation and cognitive decline may be made worse by Alzheimer's disease risk and physical activity

Bad Diet: A diet high in processed foods, saturated fats, and refined carbohydrates increases the risk of Alzheimer's disease.

The Purpose of the Mediterranean Diet:

Here's a comprehensive look at how the Mediterranean diet may impact Alzheimer's disease:

Rich in Antioxidants: Fruits, vegetables, nuts, and olive oil are all abundant in the Mediterranean diet and are rich sources of antioxidants such polyphenols and vitamins C and E. These antioxidants aid in the fight against oxidative stress, which is thought to contribute to the onset and advancement of Alzheimer's disease.

Heart Health: Because the Mediterranean diet places a strong emphasis on ingesting heart-healthy fats like those found in olive oil and fatty fish, it is well known for its heart-healthy effects. Given the strong correlation between cardiovascular and mental health, research indicates that heart health is positively correlated with brain health. A higher risk is also linked to conditions that are heart disease risk factors, such as diabetes, high cholesterol, and hypertension.

Omega-3 Fatty Acids: Fish is an excellent source of omega-3 fatty acids, especially EPA (eicosapentaenoic acid) and DHA (docosahexaenoic acid), which are essential to a Mediterranean diet. It has been demonstrated that omega-3 fatty acids possess neuroprotective qualities. They may also aid in lowering brain inflammation, which could minimize the risk of cognitive decline and Alzheimer's disease.

Low in Refined Sugars, Processed Foods, and Red Meat: Studies have shown a correlation between a higher risk of Alzheimer's disease and a Mediterranean diet that limits these three food groups. Rather, it promotes eating whole, unprocessed foods that are full of nutrients and don't include the dangerous additives that are frequently present in processed foods.

Healthy Brain Aging: According to certain research, older persons who follow a Mediterranean diet appear to have a reduced rate of cognitive decline and higher general brain health. Though further investigation is required to completely comprehend the mechanisms underlying this correlation, the Mediterranean diet's blend of nutrient-dense foods, healthful fats, and antioxidants is thought to promote ideal brain aging.

Decreased Inflammation: Alzheimer's disease is thought to be partly caused by chronic inflammation. With its focus on anti-inflammatory foods including fruits, vegetables, nuts, and fatty fish, the Mediterranean diet may help lessen inflammation in the body as a whole, including the brain.

Gut Microbiota: New research indicates that the population of bacteria that live in the digestive system, known as the gut microbiota, may be positively impacted by a Mediterranean diet. A balanced gut microbiome has been linked to improved mental and general wellness. The varied and well-balanced gut flora that is supported by the fiber-rich foods found in the Mediterranean diet—such as fruits, vegetables, and whole grains—may enhance cognitive performance.

It is crucial to remember that diet is only one aspect of the problem, even though the Mediterranean diet appears to be promising in lowering the risk of Alzheimer's disease and promoting brain health. Cognitive health and the risk of Alzheimer's disease are also significantly influenced by other factors, including heredity, physical activity, mental stimulation, and social interaction.

Symptoms and Progression of Alzheimer's Disease:

Symptoms of Alzheimer's Disease:

AD typically progresses through several stages, each characterized by distinct symptoms:

The stage known as mild cognitive impairment (MCI) is defined by slight changes in cognitive functioning, such as difficulty concentrating and forgetfulness. Although these alterations may be felt by individuals with MCI, they often have little impact on daily activities.

Early-stage Alzheimer's Disease: Symptoms worsen as the illness progresses. The severity of memory loss influences conversations and events from recently. It's possible for people to have trouble planning, organizing, and solving issues. Changes in mood and behavior, such as irritability or withdrawal, may also manifest.

Moderate Stages of Alzheimer's Disease: A more severe cognitive decline characterizes this stage. Some people may find simple tasks like dressing and taking a bath challenging. Linguistic hurdles could exist and make communication challenging. An uptick in anger and irritation are instances of behavioral signs.

Severe Alzheimer's Disease: As the condition worsens, a person's ability to perform basic daily tasks independently and effectively communicates is lost. Individuals may get very disoriented and lose their capacity to recognize loved ones. It is possible to experience physical adverse effects such as rigidity and difficulty swallowing.

Alzheimer's Disease Progression:

Although it differs from person to person, AD typically follows a recognizable pattern over time:

Initial Decline: The symptoms of AD develop gradually, often going unnoticed by the affected individual and their family. Memory loss and mild cognitive deficits could first be dismissed as normal aging symptoms.

Acceleration of Symptoms: Cognitive deterioration accelerates with worsening AD and impacts many aspects of daily life. The difficulty of routine work increases, leading to strain.

Functional Decline: Individuals with AD who are in the advanced stages of the illness have a significant functional decline and require help with daily activities such as eating, dressing, and going to the bathroom. As people become more dependent on one another, caregiver support becomes increasingly important.

Late Stages of Alzheimer's Disease: People with AD are often immobile, profoundly impaired, and verbally incapable. Malnourishment and infections are two instances of medical conditions that might arise and impair overall health.

Alzheimer's Disease and the Mediterranean Diet:

The characteristics of the Mediterranean diet include low intakes of processed foods and red meat, moderate intakes of fish and poultry, and high intakes of fruits, vegetables, whole grains, legumes, nuts, and olive oil.

A Mediterranean-Style Diet Has Been Shown to Help Prevent AD in A Number of Ways, Including:

Impact on Neuroprotection: Rich in antioxidants and anti-inflammatory compounds, the Mediterranean diet may help prevent inflammation and neuronal damage caused by AD.

Cardiovascular Health: The Mediterranean diet has been linked to improved cardiovascular health and lowered risk factors for heart disease and stroke. Given that vascular factors are associated with the development of AD, heart health may benefit brain function.

Improved Cognitive Performance: Studies have connected a Mediterranean diet to improved cognitive performance as well as a decreased risk of cognitive decline and Alzheimer's disease (AD). Omega-3 fatty acids from seafood and monounsaturated fats from olive oil are two dietary components that may support brain function.

Potential Mechanisms: One possible way that the Mediterranean Diet treats AD is by lowering oxidative stress, inflammation, and insulin resistance—all of which are connected to the disease's etiology.

Alzheimer's disease is a horrible condition that affects the patient and their family greatly. While there is currently no cure, some lifestyle decisions, such as diet, may help prevent and manage it.

The Mediterranean Diet, which emphasizes plant-based meals and healthy fats, shows promise in enhancing brain function and reducing the risk of cognitive decline associated with Alzheimer's disease. To completely understand the mechanisms underlying the effects of nutrition, more study is needed in order to prevent and treat AD.

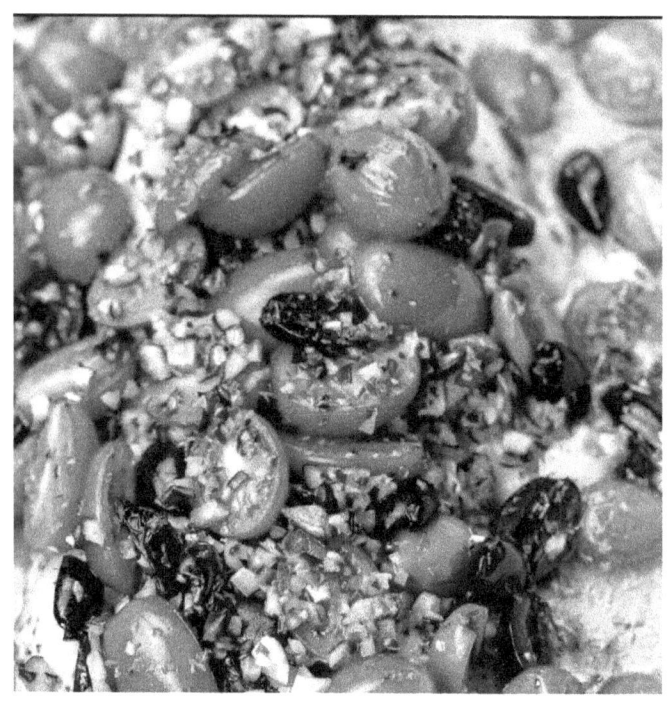

CHAPTER 2:
OVERVIEW OF THE MEDITERRANEAN DIET

Origins and History

The phrase "Mediterranean diet" was coined in the 1950s by American scientist Ancel Keys, who was observing how people in the Mediterranean region dined. However, the culinary traditions it represents date back many generations. The Mediterranean region is home to several different civilizations, including Greece, Italy, Spain, and southern France, all of which have left their own culinary legacies behind.

Essential Components of a Mediterranean Diet:

The Mediterranean diet is characterized by a high consumption of whole grains, fruits, vegetables, legumes, nuts, and olive oil. A moderate consumption of fish, poultry, and dairy products combined with a low intake of red meat and sweets are further characteristics of this eating pattern. Eating meals with loved ones, getting regular exercise, and social interaction are all highly valued aspects of the Mediterranean diet.

Historical Context and Cultural Significance:

The dietary habits of individuals residing in the Mediterranean region are influenced by their agricultural heritage and cultural practices. For millennia, the people who live around the Mediterranean coast have relied on fish, vegetables, and locally farmed olive oil as basic staples. These eating habits evolved in response to environmental and social standards, resulting in a gastronomic legacy that improves health.

Empirical Research and Alzheimer's Disease:

Numerous research works have looked into the potential benefits of the Mediterranean diet for preserving brain function, including its potential to reduce the risk of Alzheimer's disease.

Research suggests that a diet rich in antioxidants, anti-inflammatory agents, and omega-3 fatty acids may provide defense against neurodegeneration and cognitive decline. A Mediterranean diet has also been connected to a lower incidence of Alzheimer's disease and milder

Mechanisms of Action:

Numerous mechanisms may be responsible for the positive effects of a Mediterranean diet on neuroprotection.

Monounsaturated fats and polyphenols found in olive oil, the primary fat source in this diet pattern, support vascular health and reduce oxidative stress in the brain.

A diet high in fruits, vegetables, and seafood provides essential nutrients and bioactive chemicals that support brain function and synaptic plasticity, while also reducing inflammation and amyloid-beta deposition, features of Alzheimer's disease.

Future Directions and Clinical Implications:

The benefits of a Mediterranean diet for Alzheimer's disease are becoming more well recognized, and doctors are starting to incorporate dietary recommendations into their treatment plans. Cognitive impairment in at-risk persons may be prevented or delayed by therapies that support adherence to the Mediterranean diet and lifestyle modifications like physical activity and social contact.

The rich culinary heritage that is embodied by the Mediterranean diet is intricately linked to the customs and cultural practices of the Mediterranean region. Its emphasis on nutrient-dense, nutritious foods and lifestyle choices aligns with recent research demonstrating the role that diet plays in preserving brain function and reducing the risk of Alzheimer's disease.

Knowing the history and origins of the Mediterranean diet helps us better understand how useful it is for controlling and preventing Alzheimer's disease today. In addition to potential health benefits, following this eating pattern cultivates an appreciation for the lengthy history of Mediterranean cuisine.

Core Principles and Components

The Mediterranean diet must include a wide variety of fruits, vegetables, whole grains, legumes, nuts, seeds, and olive oil. This dietary pattern is characterized by a moderate amount of fish, poultry, dairy products (particularly yogurt and cheese), and red wine, along with a minimal intake of processed foods and red meat. In addition to food, the Mediterranean lifestyle emphasizes family mealtimes, regular exercise, and social contact.

Fundamental Approaches:

Plant-based Focus: The Mediterranean diet's primary focus is on plant-based foods that are rich in antioxidants, vitamins, and minerals. Berries, almonds, and leafy greens are among the nutrient-dense foods that can help combat inflammation and oxidative stress, two elements that are connected to the pathogenesis of Alzheimer's disease.

Good Fats: Olive oil is a cornerstone of the Mediterranean diet because of its high content of monounsaturated fats and phenolic compounds. These heart-healthy fats contain neuroprotective qualities that enhance cognitive function and reduce the risk of Alzheimer's disease-related cognitive decline.

Omega-3 Fatty Acids: Found in fatty fish such as salmon, mackerel, and sardines, omega-3 fatty acids are rich in eicosapentaenoic acid (EPA) and docosahexaenoic acid (DHA). These essential fatty acids maintain synaptic function and neuronal integrity, protecting against Alzheimer's-related neurodegeneration.

Moderate Wine Consumption: Red wine has drawn attention when it is incorporated into a Mediterranean diet in moderation, maybe because of its neuroprotective qualities. Resveratrol is a polyphenolic compound found in red wine that has anti-inflammatory and antioxidant properties that enhance mental health and cognitive function.

Social Engagement: In addition to culinary components, the Mediterranean lifestyle strongly emphasizes social interaction and shared meals. Engaging in purposeful social interactions fosters emotional stability, cognitive stimulation, and resilience against the progression of Alzheimer's disease.

Implications for Alzheimer's Disease Management:

The Mediterranean diet's nutrient-dense foods and lifestyle components have a lot of promise for treating Alzheimer's disease. By prioritizing brain-healthy diet and cultivating a supportive social environment, people can actively safeguard cognitive function and avoid Alzheimer's-related cognitive decline.

Furthermore, ongoing research aims to elucidate the molecular processes that underlie the Mediterranean diet's benefits, perhaps leading to customized dietary interventions for those at risk of or already suffering from Alzheimer's disease.

Health Benefits Beyond Nutrition

The Mediterranean Diet: More Than Just Food:
It is commonly known that the Mediterranean diet places a strong emphasis on whole foods while limiting processed items and red meat. Fruits, vegetables, whole grains, nuts, seeds, seafood, and olive oil are some examples of these foods.

However, its benefits go beyond nutrition alone. Several elements of the Mediterranean lifestyle promote overall health, including:

Social Engagement:

Eating together and sharing meals are highly valued in Mediterranean countries, as they foster the formation of strong social bonds. Social engagement and interaction have been shown to protect cognitive function and reduce the risk of Alzheimer's disease.

Physical Activity:

Frequent physical activity, such as walking, gardening, and casually playing board games, is an important part of the Mediterranean diet. Exercise has been shown to boost brain health by increasing neuroplasticity and reducing the risk of cognitive decline.

Stress Reduction:

Carefree Mediterranean lifestyles frequently prioritize relaxation techniques like yoga, mindfulness, and outdoor pursuits. Because stress has been linked to cognitive impairment and may exacerbate the pathology of the disease, it is crucial for both prevention and therapy of Alzheimer's disease.

Adequate Sleep:

Adequate sleep is essential for mental and cognitive health. Getting a good night's sleep is often highly valued in Mediterranean cultures, where sleep routines are followed and calming activities are done directly before bed.

Alzheimer's Disease and The Mediterranean Diet:

Anti-inflammatory Effects:

The Mediterranean diet, which is rich in anti-inflammatory foods like fruits, vegetables, and olive oil, minimizes pro-inflammatory foods like processed foods and trans fats. Chronic inflammation is linked to the etiology of Alzheimer's disease; therefore, a diet rich in anti-inflammatory foods may help reduce neuroinflammation and reduce the risk of cognitive decline.

Antioxidant Protection:

Plant-based foods that are rich in antioxidants make up a significant element of the Mediterranean diet. These foods aid in the prevention of oxidative stress and the neutralization of free radicals that harm neurons. Due to its high antioxidant content, the Mediterranean diet may help protect against the oxidative damage associated with Alzheimer's disease.

Brain-Healthy Nutrients:

A number of nutrients, such as omega-3 fatty acids from fish, polyphenols from fruits and vegetables, and vitamin E from nuts and seeds, are abundant in the Mediterranean diet and have been shown to enhance cognitive function and brain health. These nutrients may enhance synaptic plasticity, increase cerebral blood flow, and trigger neurogenesis—all critical processes for preserving cognitive function and reducing the risk of Alzheimer's disease.

In addition to its nutritional benefits, the Mediterranean diet fosters social, physical, and psychological well-being—all of which are critical for both managing and preventing Alzheimer's disease. In addition to enjoying delicious and nourishing meals, those who follow the Mediterranean diet may be able to reduce their risk of cognitive decline and enhance their overall quality of life.

Changing to a Mediterranean diet and lifestyle offers a practical means of promoting brain health and combating the increasing incidence of Alzheimer's disease.

Scientific Proof of Its Effectiveness

A lowered risk of heart disease, cancer, and neurological conditions like AD are just a few of the health advantages of this dietary pattern. It is fashioned around the customary eating patterns of Mediterranean Sea.

Reduced Risk of Cognitive Decline:

Numerous observational studies have shown that adhering to a Mediterranean diet is consistently associated with a decreased incidence of dementia and cognitive decline, including AD.

A prospective cohort study published in the journal Neurology found a correlation between shorter cognitive decline in older adults and stronger adherence to the Mediterranean diet over a 4-year follow-up period. Another long-term study indicated that older people with moderate cognitive impairment (MCI) and incident AD were less likely to follow a Mediterranean diet (published in JAMA Internal Medicine).

Neuroprotective Effects:

Foods abundant in antioxidants, such fatty fish, fruits, and vegetables, have neuroprotective properties that may help preserve cognitive function and reduce the incidence of

AD.

The polyphenols found in red wine and olive oil have been shown to have anti-inflammatory and antioxidant effects in the brain.

This suggests that they may reduce neuro-inflammation and oxidative stress, two elements associated with the development of Alzheimer's disease. Omega-3 fatty acids, which are abundant in fish like salmon and mackerel and have anti-inflammatory and neuroprotective properties, have been linked to improved cognitive performance and a decreased risk of Alzheimer's disease.

Impact on Brain Structure and Function:

Recent studies have used neuroimaging techniques, such as magnetic resonance imaging (MRI) and positron emission tomography (PET), to shed insight on how the Mediterranean diet affects the structure and function of the brain.

A Mediterranean diet has been associated with increased gray matter and total brain sizes, which are indicators of better brain health and a decreased risk of neurodegeneration, according to a Neurology study.

A second investigation that was published in the Journal of Alzheimer's Disease found that those who ate a Mediterranean-style diet had lower levels of beta-amyloid plaques, a pathology that is typical of AD. According to this research, a Mediterranean diet may help prevent the accumulation of amyloid.

The Mediterranean diet is a useful nutritional approach for reducing the risk of Alzheimer's and preserving cognitive function in older adults. This dietary pattern has been shown in studies to have favorable effects on brain structure and function, neuroprotective qualities, and a lower risk of cognitive decline.

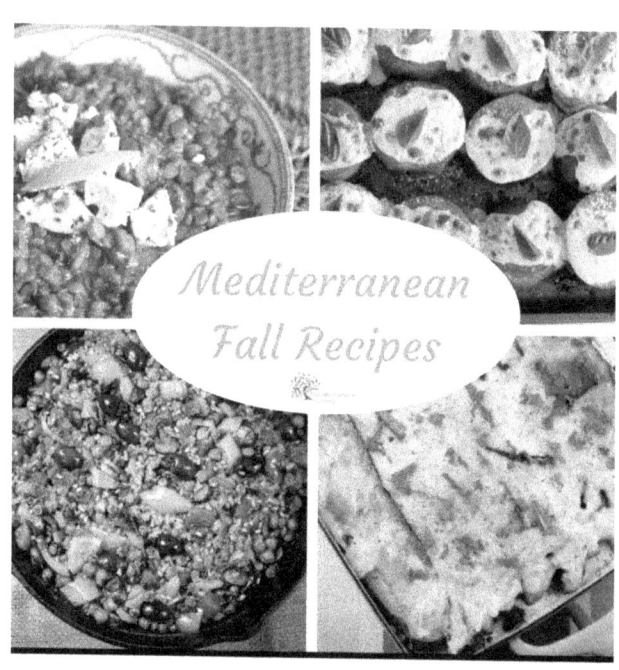

Mediterranean Fall Recipes

CHAPTER 3:
NUTRITIONAL FOUNDATIONS OF THE MEDITERRANEAN DIET

Emphasis on Plant-Based Foods

The plant-based diet is the cornerstone of the Mediterranean diet. These foods offer neuroprotective and anti-inflammatory properties that are essential for brain function.

They are also rich in antioxidants, vitamins, minerals, and phytochemicals. Berries, oranges, and grapes are rich in flavonoids and vitamin C, which help combat oxidative stress and inflammation, two important factors associated with the progression of Alzheimer's disease.

Foods high in essential nutrients like carotenoids, vitamin K, and folate, which enhance cognitive function and reduce the incidence of cognitive decline, include tomatoes, leafy greens, and cruciferous vegetables.

The Role of Olive Oil:

Olive oil, an essential component of the Mediterranean diet, merits particular consideration due to its neuroprotective qualities. Rich in monounsaturated fats and polyphenols, olive oil contains anti-inflammatory and antioxidant qualities that shield brain tissue from damage. Since consuming it has been linked to improved memory and cognitive function, it is a helpful strategy in the prevention of Alzheimer's disease.

Nuts, Legumes, and Whole Grains:

Nuts, legumes, and whole grains are mainstays of the Mediterranean diet and offer a host of health benefits. Nuts like pistachios, walnuts, and almonds that are high in antioxidants, vitamin E, and omega-3 fatty acids promote brain health and reduce the risk of cognitive decline.

Legumes, including beans, lentils, and chickpeas, are high in fiber, protein, and vitamins and help support a healthy brain. Whole grains including oats, brown rice, and quinoa provide sustained energy and enhance cognitive resilience.

Fish and Poultry:

The Mediterranean diet is mostly plant-based, but it also includes moderate amounts of fish and fowl, which provide vital elements to the overall pattern. Rich sources of omega-3 fatty acids include fatty fish like mackerel, sardines, and salmon. These Fats are essential for mental and cognitive function. Poultry provides high-quality protein and B vitamins, which are important for the synthesis of neurotransmitters and cognitive function. This is especially true with lean cuts.

Plant-based foods can be included in the Mediterranean diet as part of a complete strategy to prevent Alzheimer's disease. People can improve their cognitive performance and reduce the risk of cognitive decline by consuming fruits, vegetables, nuts, legumes, whole grains, and olive oil. Changing one's eating habits to this one fosters physical and mental health, allowing a healthier you.

Role of Healthy Fats and Oils:

Monounsaturated and polyunsaturated fats, which are very beneficial fats, are abundant in the Mediterranean diet. These fats are essential for maintaining the structural integrity of cell membranes, reducing inflammation, and facilitating nerve transmission.

Olive oil, which is rich in monounsaturated fats and antioxidants like oleocanthal and oleuropein that have neuroprotective and anti-inflammatory properties, is a crucial part of the Mediterranean diet.

Another key component of the Mediterranean diet is omega-3 fatty acids, which are mostly found in fatty fish like salmon, sardines, and mackerel. These fats—docosahexaenoic acid (DHA) and eicosapentaenoic acid (EPA) in particular—are critical for brain function, neuroplasticity, and reducing the risk of cognitive decline. Additionally, the anti-inflammatory qualities of omega-3s may reduce neuro inflammation associated with the etiology of Alzheimer's disease.

Impact on Alzheimer's Disease:

An increasing body of research indicates that older adults who consume a Mediterranean-style diet are less likely to develop Alzheimer's disease and their rate of cognitive decline is also slower. There are several mechanisms underlying these protective effects:

Diminishment of Oxidative Stress: The antioxidants included in olive oil and other foods from the Mediterranean diet operate as a defense against free radicals, thereby reducing oxidative stress, which has been connected to the progression of Alzheimer's disease.

Anti-Inflammatory Properties: The polyphenols and omega-3 fatty acids found in olive oil possess potent anti-inflammatory properties that can mitigate neuro inflammation and diminish the likelihood of developing Alzheimer's disease.

Maintenance of Vascular Health: Heart health, which in turn supports adequate blood flow to the brain, is a crucial aspect of the Mediterranean diet, which reduces the prevalence of vascular dementia, a significant co-morbidity of Alzheimer's disease.

Promotion of Neuroplasticity: Omega-3 fatty acids are essential for maintaining synaptic plasticity, protecting the structure and function of neurons, and enhancing cognitive performance throughout life.

In a nutshell including healthy fats and oils in the Mediterranean diet may help reduce the risk of Alzheimer's disease and preserve cognitive function in older populations. People who emphasize foods rich in monounsaturated fats, omega-3 fatty acids, and antioxidants can benefit from the neuroprotective advantages of this dietary pattern.

Moderate Consumption of Fish and Poultry

Fish, particularly fatty fish like salmon, mackerel, and sardines, is an excellent source of omega-3 fatty acids, particularly EPA (eicosapentaenoic acid) and DHA (docosahexaenoic acid). The manufacture of neurotransmitters, preservation of the integrity of neuronal membranes, and stimulation of neuroplasticity in the brain all depend on these crucial fatty acids.

According to research, eating fish regularly is associated with a decreased risk of Alzheimer's disease and cognitive decline. This association may be due to fish's anti-inflammatory and neuroprotective properties.

Poultry: A Lean Protein Source for Brain Health:

Poultry products, such chicken and turkey, are commended for having a high lean protein content and a low saturated fat profile. Protein is necessary for the synthesis of neurotransmitters as well as the maintenance of brain tissue. Vitamin B12, which is necessary for healthy nerves and cognitive function, is also abundant in poultry.

When incorporated into a well-balanced diet such as the Mediterranean diet, poultry can still enhance general brain health and cognitive performance, even though its association with Alzheimer's disease has not attracted as much attention as that of fish consumption.

Moderation is Key:

Even though fish and poultry provide helpful elements for brain health, moderation is still important. Certain fish species, such as those high in mercury, might be dangerous to your health if consumed in excess. Additionally, some methods of meal preparation, such frying, can negate the nutritional benefits of specific meals.

It is also essential to prioritize grilled, baked, or steamed preparations and to diversify the types of fish and poultry consumed in order to optimize benefits and minimize risks.

The Mediterranean diet stands out in the hunt for Alzheimer's disease treatment therapies and preventive measures because it is a holistic approach that blends delicious food with major health benefits. Fish and poultry in moderation offer vital nutrients that support brain function and may help reduce the risk of cognitive decline when incorporated into this eating pattern.

Combining the principles of the Mediterranean diet with other health-conscious lifestyle decisions may help prevent Alzheimer's and offer promise for a better, more cognitively resilient future.

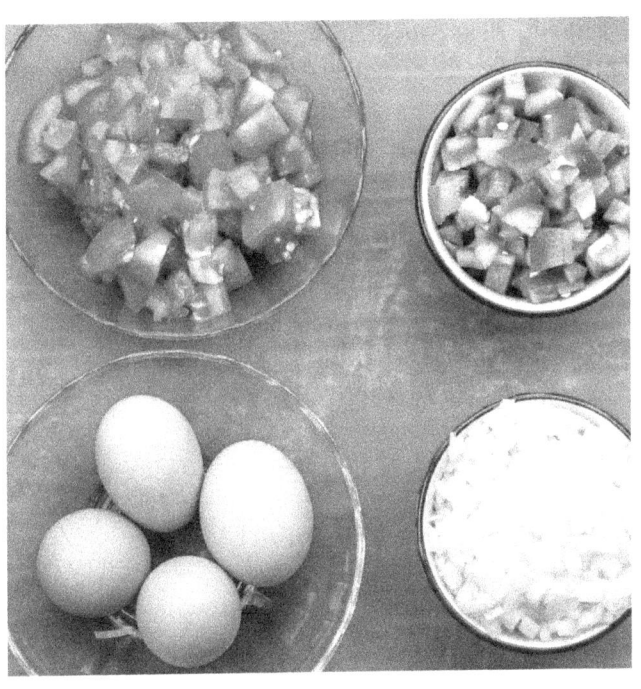

Limited Red Meat and Processed Foods

Overindulgence in red meat eating has been connected to certain health risks, such as type 2 diabetes, cardiovascular disease, and specific cancers. Studies have suggested a possible link between a high red meat intake and an increased risk of cognitive decline in the setting of Alzheimer's disease.

This correlation may be explained by a number of factors, including oxidative stress, inflammation, and the accumulation of amyloid-beta plaques in the brain—all of which are hallmarks of the pathology connected to Alzheimer's disease.

Processed Foods and Cognitive Health:

Because processed foods are loaded with unhealthy fats, refined sugars, and additives, they are a regular sight in diets today. Eating processed food frequently may exacerbate cognitive decline and increase the risk of Alzheimer's disease, according to a growing body of evidence. These detrimental effects are thought to be caused by the pro-inflammatory and oxidative properties of several food additives, as well as by their detrimental impact on insulin sensitivity and metabolic health.

The Protective Role of the Mediterranean Diet:

Contrary to the harmful effects of red meat and processed foods, the Mediterranean diet offers a wealth of minerals and bioactive compounds with neuroprotective characteristics. Rich in vitamins, minerals, omega-3 fatty acids, and antioxidants, this dietary pattern supports healthy brain function, reduces inflammation, and combats oxidative stress. Vascular dementia is a common co-morbidity of Alzheimer's disease that can be avoided by consuming plant-based diets high in healthy fats and nutrients that promote cardiovascular health.

Practical Recommendations:

Integrating the principles of the Mediterranean diet into daily life can be a practical and effective strategy for preventing Alzheimer's. Among the specific measures are:

Prioritize plant-based foods: Plant-based foods should take precedence over other foods. Fill your plate with an abundance of colorful fruits, vegetables, legumes, and complete grains.

Choose your lean protein sources: Choose fish, poultry, and plant-based proteins like beans and lentils over red meat. Accept healthy fats: Include avocados, almonds, and seeds in your diet, and get the majority of your fat from olive oil.

Cut back on the quantity of processed foods: Limit your intake of pre-made meals, sugary beverages, and packaged snacks in favor of complete, less processed foods.

Savor meals with loved ones: In addition to its nutritional benefits, the Mediterranean diet encourages social interactions and mindful eating, which both enhance overall wellbeing and cognitive health.

The health advantages of fresh produce, legumes, and whole grains

A Mediterranean diet must include fresh produce because it is a fantastic source of vitamins, minerals, and antioxidants. It is the diet's main component. Lowering oxidative stress and inflammation—two factors that are known to play a big role in the development of Alzheimer's disease—is made possible by these nutrients. Studies have shown time and time again that a diet rich in fresh produce lowers the risk of cognitive decline and the onset of Alzheimer's disease.

Whole Grains for Brain Health:

Because of their high fiber content and complex carbohydrates, whole grains like quinoa, brown rice, barley, and oats are vital components of the Mediterranean diet. These nutrients provide a steady stream of glucose to the brain, supporting optimal cognitive function.

Moreover, whole grains are an excellent source of B vitamins, including folate, which has been linked to a decreased risk of cognitive decline and Alzheimer's disease. By incorporating whole grains into their daily meals, people can improve their brain function and lower their risk of developing neurodegenerative disorders.

The Power of Legumes:

Beans, lentils, and chickpeas are examples of legumes, which are nutrient-dense foods that are high in fiber, protein, and essential vitamins and minerals. When they are included in the Mediterranean diet, there are numerous benefits for brain health.

Legumes help to maintain consistent energy levels, which are necessary for optimal brain function and to avoid blood sugar spikes, because they have a low glycemic index. The high folate content of legumes may also reduce the risk of Alzheimer's disease while maintaining cognitive function. Regular bean consumption has been associated with improved memory, concentration, and brain health.

An effective strategy in the fight against Alzheimer's disease seems to be a Mediterranean diet rich in fresh fruit, whole grains, and legumes. In addition to giving the body sustenance, these dietary components guard against neurodegenerative diseases and preserve cognitive function.

Adopting the principles of the Mediterranean diet can help people actively protect their brain health and enhance their general well-being. Per the adage "Let food be thy medicine," a Mediterranean diet can improve one's mind and future while also acting as a potent cure for Alzheimer's disease.

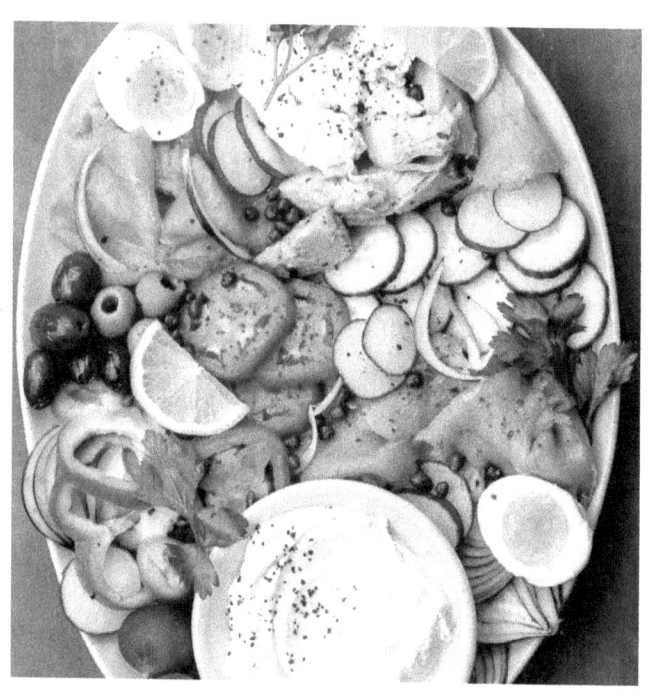

CHAPTER 4: MEDITERRANEAN DIET AND BRAIN HEALTH

Mechanisms Behind Diet-Brain Connection

The cornerstone of the Mediterranean diet is consuming plant-based foods including fruits, vegetables, whole grains, legumes, nuts, and olive oil together with a modest quantity of dairy, red wine, fish, and poultry. The abundance of antioxidants, polyphenols, omega-3 fatty acids, and other bioactive ingredients in this diet plan is widely known. Together, these compounds protect the heart, lower inflammation, and may even maintain cognitive function.

Mechanisms Linking Diet to Brain Function:

Anti-inflammatory Effects: It is believed that long-term inflammation is the root cause of Alzheimer's disease. The Mediterranean diet helps lower neuro inflammation, which lowers neuronal damage and preserves cognitive function since it is rich in antioxidants and anti-inflammatory substances.

Antioxidant Properties: Oxidative stress, a key component in the pathogenesis of AD, produces reactive oxygen species (ROS) and neuronal damage. The high antioxidant content of the Mediterranean diet shields brain cells from free radical damage and prevents oxidative damage.

Neuroprotection via Omega-3 Fatty Acids: Particularly the fatty acids eicosapentaenoic acid (EPA) and docosahexaenoic acid (DHA), which are present in fatty fish, exhibit neuroprotective effects and lower the risk of developing Alzheimer's disease (AD) by enhancing synaptic function, reducing neuro inflammation, and promoting the removal of amyloid-beta peptides.

Gut Microbiota Regulation: Emerging research points to a "gut-brain axis," or reciprocal relationship, between gut microbiota and brain health. The Mediterranean diet, which is high in fiber and prebiotics, helps to create a diverse and beneficial gut flora, which in turn influences the synthesis of neurotransmitters, the generation of neurotrophic factor, and neuro inflammation—all of which are connected to the pathophysiology of AD.

Clinical Guidance and Future Directions:

A number of epidemiological studies and clinical trials have highlighted the benefits of the Mediterranean diet in averting Alzheimer's disease and cognitive decline. Further research is required to elucidate the optimal dietary components, adherence levels, and long-term effects on the lowering of AD risk.

The complex relationship between nutrition and brain health opens up new possibilities for managing and preventing Alzheimer's disease. Adopting the Mediterranean diet's tenets, which are known for their anti-inflammatory, antioxidant, neuroprotective, and microbiota-modulating qualities, can enable people to protect their cognitive function and maintain brain vibrancy far into old life.

The integration of dietary treatments into comprehensive approaches for the prevention of AD remains a crucial need in global public health programs, as research endeavors to unravel the mechanisms behind the diet-brain relationship.

Research on Mediterranean Diet and Brain Health

Many studies have examined the relationship between eating a Mediterranean diet and many aspects of brain health. According to studies, those who follow this eating pattern exhibit the following behaviors:

Reduced Cognitive Decline: Studies utilizing observational data have consistently shown that older adults who consume a Mediterranean diet experience less cognitive decline. A meta-analysis that was published in the journal Epidemiology found that strong adherence to the Mediterranean diet was associated with a 30% decreased risk of cognitive impairment.

Lower Risk of Alzheimer's Disease: A Mediterranean diet has been linked to a lower risk of Alzheimer's disease, per a number of studies. A study that was published in the journal Alzheimer's & Dementia found that those who ate a Mediterranean diet had a 33% lower risk of developing Alzheimer's disease (AD) than those who did not.

Preserving Brain Structure: Studies on neuroimaging have provided insight into the benefits of a Mediterranean diet for maintaining brain structure. According to research published in the journal Neurology, adhering to this dietary pattern was associated with both an increased overall brain volume and better preservation of gray matter volume in brain regions crucial for memory and cognition.

Mechanisms of Action:

The favorable effects of the Mediterranean diet on brain health may be mediated through a variety of different pathways.

Anti-inflammatory Properties: The abundance of fruits, vegetables, and olive oil in the diet has anti-inflammatory properties that may mitigate neuro inflammation, a condition linked to Alzheimer's disease.

Antioxidant Activity: The oxidative stress that is connected to the genesis of AD is averted by following a Mediterranean diet rich in antioxidants such as vitamin E, flavonoids, and polyphenols.

Cardiovascular Health: Given the strong association between heart health and brain function, it is expected that the Mediterranean diet's beneficial effects on heart health will also indirectly improve cognitive performance and reduce the risk of neurodegenerative disorders.

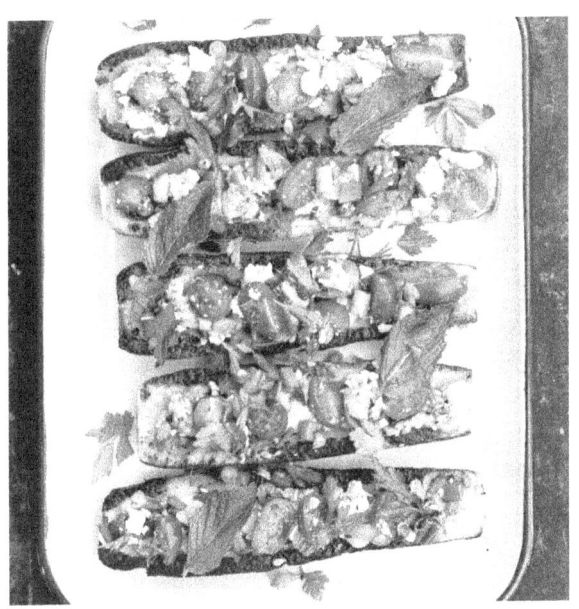

Implications for the Management of Alzheimer's Disease: Although more research is needed to fully understand the role of the Mediterranean diet in managing and preventing Alzheimer's disease, it may be employed as a therapy intervention.

Integrating elements of the Mediterranean diet with lifestyle interventions may offer a multimodal approach to slowing cognitive decline and improving quality of life for individuals with AD or at risk of getting the condition.

The Mediterranean diet is one dietary strategy that has shown promise for promoting cognitive function and maybe lowering the risk of Alzheimer's disease. Its emphasis on wholesome, nutrient-dense foods aligns with the principles of good aging and may offer a practical and enjoyable way to preserve cognitive abilities.

Additional investigation into the mechanisms underlying its benefits and efficacy as an adjuvant therapy for AD is necessary to fully realize its promise in the treatment of neurodegenerative illnesses. Eating a Mediterranean diet feeds the mind in addition to the body, offering a holistic approach to maintaining cognitive health throughout life.

Potential Benefits for Alzheimer's Disease Prevention and Management

Renowned for emphasizing whole grains, fruits, vegetables, nuts, olive oil, and fish, the Mediterranean diet has shown encouraging results in treating a number of illnesses, such as cognitive decline and cardiovascular disease. We examine the possible advantages of the Mediterranean diet for managing and preventing Alzheimer's disease in this thorough investigation.

Rich in Nutrients Components:

The Mediterranean diet is characterized by nutrient-dense foods that are abundant in vitamins, minerals, and antioxidants.
For instance, olive oil's monounsaturated fats and polyphenols offer neuroprotective and anti-inflammatory qualities.
Omega-3 fatty acid-rich fish is associated with improved cognitive function and a decreased risk of cognitive decline.

Anti-inflammatory Properties:

Chronic inflammation is implicated in the pathogenesis of Alzheimer's disease.

The Mediterranean diet's anti-inflammatory properties, which could potentially lessen neuroinflammation, are ascribed to its focus on fruits, vegetables, and olive oil. Polyphenols found in fruits, vegetables, and red wine have anti-inflammatory qualities that prevent neuronal damage.

Heart Health:

Cardiovascular risk factors like hypertension and dyslipidemia have been linked to an increased risk of Alzheimer's disease. Almonds, fatty salmon, and whole grains are among the heart-healthy foods featured in the

Mediterranean diet that enhance cardiovascular health and reduce the incidence of Alzheimer's disease.

Blood Sugar Regulation:

Dysregulated glucose metabolism is associated to the development of Alzheimer's disease and cognitive impairment. The Mediterranean diet's emphasis on complex carbohydrates, high-fiber meals, and limitation in alcohol use may help regulate blood sugar levels and lower the risk of Alzheimer's disease.

Regulation of Gut Microbiota:

There appears to be a connection between brain function and the composition of the gut flora.

The Mediterranean diet, which is high in fiber, probiotics, and prebiotics, fosters a beneficial and diverse gut microbiota that may enhance cognitive function and reduce the risk of Alzheimer's disease.

Social and Lifestyle Factors:

In addition to food, the Mediterranean diet incorporates social and lifestyle elements like exercise, group meals, and stress reduction.

Social engagement and mental stimulation seen in the Mediterranean lifestyle improve cognitive resilience and may even prevent cognitive loss associated with Alzheimer's disease.

The Mediterranean diet offers a wide variety of nutrient-dense foods with anti-inflammatory, cardiovascular, and neuroprotective qualities, making it a versatile approach to controlling and preventing Alzheimer's disease. Although more research is required to determine the precise causes and optimal dietary patterns, a Mediterranean-style eating pattern is a promising strategy in the battle against Alzheimer's disease.

A Mediterranean diet and other lifestyle modifications can enhance brain function, increase quality of life, and decrease the effects of Alzheimer's on both individuals and society.

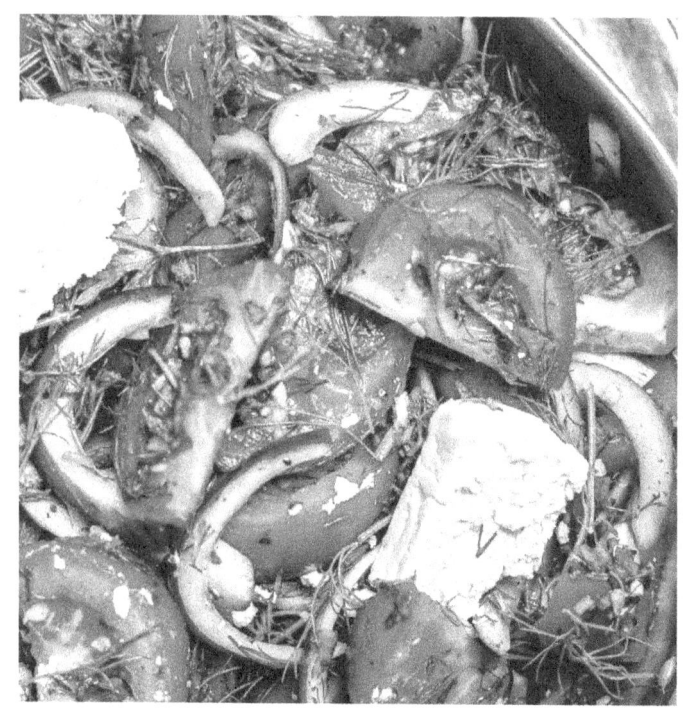

CHAPTER 5:

ANTI-INFLAMMATORY PROPERTIES OF THE MEDITERRANEAN DIET

Impact of Diet on Inflammatory Processes

These degenerative changes trigger inflammatory responses that include the activation of immune cells called microglia and astrocytes that reside in the central nervous system. While the brain's natural defense against injury and infection is inflammation, chronic inflammation can exacerbate neuronal damage and hasten the onset of Alzheimer's disease.

Role of Diet in Modulating Inflammatory Processes:

Diet plays a major role in controlling inflammation throughout the body, including the brain. Certain dietary components have been shown to either enhance or decrease inflammation, which has an impact on the risk and severity of Alzheimer's disease.

For instance, diets heavy in saturated fats and refined carbohydrates have been linked to increased inflammation and oxidative stress, two factors that are crucial to the pathogenesis of Alzheimer's disease. Conversely, a Mediterranean-style diet high in fruits, vegetables, whole grains, fish, and healthy fats like olive oil has been associated with lower levels of inflammation and a lower risk of cognitive impairment.

Key Dietary Factors and Their Impact on Alzheimer's-Related Inflammation:

Omega-3 Fatty Acids: Rich in nuts, seeds, and fatty fish, omega-3 fatty acids contain anti-inflammatory properties that may reduce neuronal inflammation in Alzheimer's patients.

Antioxidants: Flavonoids, vitamin C, and vitamin E-rich fruits and vegetables might fight oxidative stress and inflammation, which may delay the beginning of Alzheimer's disease.

Polyphenols: Rich in polyphenols, foods like berries, dark chocolate, and green tea have anti-inflammatory qualities and may protect against the neurodegeneration caused by Alzheimer's disease.

Curcumin: A component of turmeric, curcumin has shown potent anti-inflammatory and neuroprotective properties, indicating potential use in the treatment of Alzheimer's disease.

Practical Dietary Recommendations for Alzheimer's Prevention and Management:

Emphasize the advantages of a plant-based diet rich in whole grains, legumes, fruits, and vegetables because these foods provide a range of nutrients that can help lower inflammation.

Include foods like walnuts, salmon, and flaxseeds that are high in omega-3 fatty acids in your diet on a regular basis.

Processed meals, sugary snacks, and red meat should be consumed in moderation because they cause inflammation and increase the risk of Alzheimer's disease.

Consume a diet rich in antioxidant-rich foods, such as berries, leafy greens, nuts, and seeds, to combat oxidative stress.

If you would like to benefit from turmeric's potential anti-inflammatory qualities, see a physician before consuming curcumin-containing tablets or utilizing turmeric in cooking.

The relationship between diet and inflammatory processes in Alzheimer's disease is intricate and dynamic. People may be able to reduce their risk of Alzheimer's disease and slow its progression by adopting a diet that is strong in anti-inflammatory components and low in pro-inflammatory items.

However, further research is needed to identify the specific food ingredients and mechanisms underlying this complex interplay. A proactive approach to maintain cognitive function and lower the inflammatory processes associated with Alzheimer's disease is to make informed eating choices in the interim.

Foods Rich in Anti-inflammatory Compounds

Two features of brain inflammation, or neuro inflammation, which can damage neurons and impair cognitive function, are the release of pro-inflammatory chemicals and the activation of immune cells.

Fatty Fish: Omega-3 fatty acids, particularly EPA and DHA, which have potent anti-inflammatory properties, are abundant in fatty fish, including salmon, mackerel, and sardines. These essential fatty acids may improve cognitive function, reduce inflammation in the brain, and lower the risk of Alzheimer's disease.

Berries: Packed with anti-inflammatory and neuroprotective flavonoids and anthocyanins, blueberries, strawberries, raspberries, and other brightly colored berries are an excellent source of nourishment. Regular berry consumption has been associated with improved memory and cognitive function.

Leafy Green Vegetables: Collard greens, spinach, kale, and other leafy greens are rich in vitamins, minerals, and phytonutrients that help to reduce inflammation. They contain nutrients including lutein, zeaxanthin, and vitamin K that have been linked to a decreased risk of cognitive decline and Alzheimer's disease.

Nuts and Seeds: Almonds, walnuts, flaxseeds, and chia seeds are good sources of alpha-linolenic acid (ALA), a plant-based omega-3 fatty acid. Together with magnesium, vitamin E, and antioxidants, these foods also contain it. These nutrients reduce inflammation and oxidative stress in the brain, which promotes neuronal health and cognitive performance.

Turmeric: Curcumin, the main component of turmeric, has potent anti-inflammatory and antioxidant properties. Studies suggest that curcumin may reduce neuro inflammation and stop beta-amyloid plaques from forming, perhaps delaying the onset of Alzheimer's disease.
Well-known for its anti-inflammatory properties, extra virgin olive oil is a staple of the Mediterranean diet. It contains monounsaturated fats, polyphenols, and oleocanthal, which help reduce inflammation in the brain and prevent cognitive decline.

Dark Chocolate: Has a lot of cocoa Epicatechin, one of the several flavonoids found in dark chocolate, has anti-inflammatory and neuroprotective qualities. Dark chocolate can improve brain function and reduce the risk of Alzheimer's disease when ingested in moderation.

While a diet cannot prevent Alzheimer's disease on its own, incorporating anti-inflammatory foods into your meals can help preserve brain function and reduce the likelihood that you will experience cognitive loss.

By concentrating on a balanced diet rich in these foods, people can use the anti-inflammatory qualities of fatty fish, berries, leafy greens, nuts, seeds, olive oil, dark chocolate, and turmeric to feed their brains and possibly minimize the symptoms of Alzheimer's disease.

How Mediterranean Diet May Help Reduce Inflammation

Antioxidants, polyphenols, omega-3 fatty acids, and other bioactive substances with anti-inflammatory qualities abound in this dietary pattern.

Reducing Inflammatory Biomarkers:

A number of studies have demonstrated a correlation between a Mediterranean diet and lower blood levels of inflammatory biomarkers, such as C-reactive protein (CRP) and interleukin-6 (IL-6). By reducing systemic inflammation, the Mediterranean diet may mitigate the inflammatory cascade that hastens the onset of Alzheimer's disease.

Preserving Brain Health:

Research has shown that the abundance of nutrients in the Mediterranean diet enhance mental wellness and performance. For example, omega-3 fatty acids, which are typically found in fish, have anti-inflammatory qualities that may help preserve cognitive function. In addition, polyphenols, which are present in fruits, vegetables, and olive oil, have neuroprotective properties and the capacity to modify signaling pathways associated with inflammation and neurodegeneration.

Modulating Gut Microbiota:

It is possible that the Mediterranean diet influences the composition and diversity of the gut microbiota, which is critical for regulating inflammation and the immune system. This is suggested by recent research. Maintaining the integrity of the gut barrier and reducing the translocation of inflammatory molecules into the bloodstream are two ways that a healthy gut microbiota may help reduce the systemic inflammation associated with Alzheimer's disease.

With no known treatment for Alzheimer's disease, dietary therapy such as the Mediterranean diet may offer potential benefits in reducing inflammation and slowing the illness's progression. It is recommended to incorporate a variety of foods that are high in nutrients and to highlight elements that reduce inflammation in order to support cognitive function and reduce the risk of Alzheimer's disease.

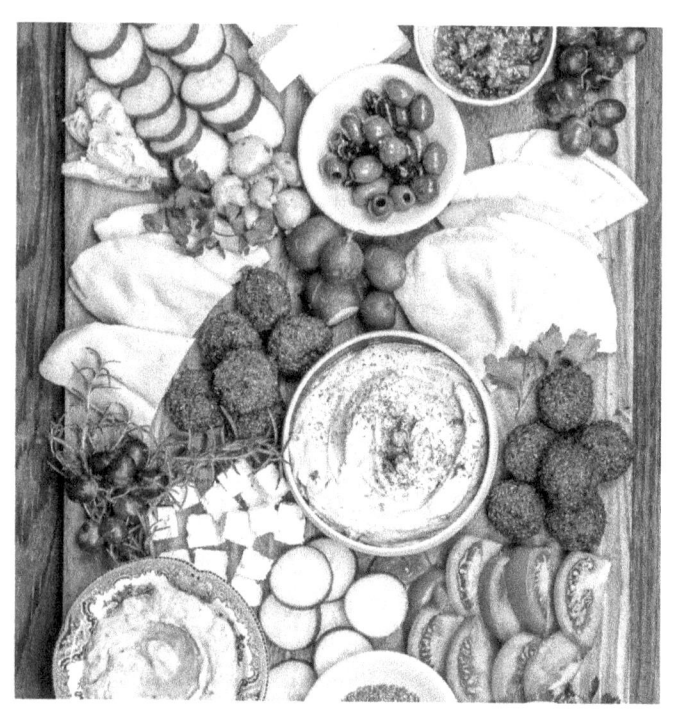

CHAPTER 6: ANTIOXIDANTS AND NEUROPROTECTION

Oxidative Stress and Neurodegeneration.

Oxidative stress is the result of an imbalance between the production of reactive oxygen species (ROS) and the ability of cells to detoxify or repair the damage they have caused. Examples of ROS that are naturally occurring byproducts of biological metabolism include superoxide, hydrogen peroxide, and hydroxyl radicals.

Free radicals (ROS) are naturally opposed by defense mechanisms in cells, which help maintain redox equilibrium. However, Alzheimer's disease throws this equilibrium off, leading to an overabundance of reactive oxygen species (ROS) and oxidative damage to cellular components such proteins, lipids, and nucleic acids.

The Part Oxidative Stress Plays in Alzheimer's Disability

In the context of Alzheimer's disease, oxidative stress is directly linked to the clinical characteristics of the condition, particularly the accumulation of amyloid-beta (Aβ) plaques and tau protein tangles in the brain.

The peptide Aβ, which is produced from the amyloid precursor protein (APP), has been shown to induce oxidative stress in multiple ways. In addition to impairing mitochondrial activity and causing direct oxidative damage, it can also activate microglia, which releases pro-inflammatory cytokines and exacerbates oxidative damage.

On the other hand, tau proteins' main job is to keep neuronal microtubules stable. In Alzheimer's disease, neurofibrillary tangles (NFTs) and compromised neuronal function are caused by hyper phosphorylation of tau. Oxidative stress prolongs tau hyper phosphorylation by activating kinases and inactivating phosphatases involved in de tau regulation.

Consequences of Oxidative Stress in Alzheimer's Disease

Oxidative stress affects Alzheimer's disease in several ways that go beyond the simple breakdown of cellular components. Oxidative stress-induced lipid peroxidation produces toxic lipid peroxides, which exacerbate inflammation and brain damage.

Protein oxidation causes structural and functional alterations in key brain proteins, interfering with signaling cascades and synaptic transmission. Moreover, genomic instability and mutations brought on by oxidative DNA damage have the potential to harm neurons and kill cells.

Therapeutic Strategies Targeting Oxidative Stress

Treatment strategies that aim to lessen oxidative damage have drawn a lot of attention since oxidative stress is a major factor in Alzheimer's disease. Antioxidants, such as vitamins C and E, have been investigated for their potential neuroprotective qualities, despite the mixed results of clinical research.

Other tactics include concentrating on the upstream causes of oxidative stress, including as Aβ aggregation and mitochondrial dysfunction, and bolstering endogenous antioxidant defense mechanisms through pharmacological or lifestyle interventions.

Oxidative stress is one of the primary processes underlying the neurodegeneration associated with Alzheimer's disease. The degenerative progression of the disease is tightly linked to the interplay between ROS production, cellular damage, and antioxidant defenses. Understanding the molecular pathways of oxidative stress in Alzheimer's disease is crucial to developing novel therapeutic approaches aimed at halting or slowing the disease's progression.

Mediterranean-Style Dietary Supplements

Antioxidants protect cells from oxidative stress by neutralizing reactive oxygen species (ROS) and reducing oxidative stress. In the context of Alzheimer's disease, antioxidants are crucial for minimizing neuronal damage and preserving cognitive function. Research has shown that an antioxidant-rich diet can reduce the incidence of AD and slow the disease's progression by reducing oxidative damage, lowering inflammation, and promoting neuroplasticity.

Key Antioxidant-Rich Components of the Mediterranean Diet:

Extra Virgin Olive Oil: Extra virgin olive oil has potent anti-inflammatory and antioxidant properties due to its high content of phenolic compounds and oleic acid. Olive oil use as part of a Mediterranean diet has been associated with a decreased risk of Alzheimer's disease and cognitive decline.

Fruits and Vegetables: A wonderful source of nourishment, colorful fruits and vegetables are high in vitamins, minerals, and phytochemicals that have antioxidant properties. Berries, citrus fruits, leafy greens, and tomatoes are particularly rich sources of antioxidants, including vitamin C, flavonoids, and carotenoids. These foods are often included in a Mediterranean diet.

Nuts and Seeds: Packed full of vitamin E, selenium, and polyphenols, nuts and seeds are a great source of antioxidants. Almonds, walnuts, and flaxseeds are three staples of the Mediterranean diet that have been linked to improved cognitive function and a decreased risk of AD.

Fish: Rich sources of neuroprotective and anti-inflammatory omega-3 fatty acids are fatty fish like mackerel, salmon, and sardines. Frequent fish consumption as part of a Mediterranean diet has been associated with a lower risk of Alzheimer's disease and cognitive decline.

The Mediterranean diet has great promise for controlling and possibly preventing Alzheimer's disease because it emphasizes foods high in antioxidants. Since they lessen oxidative stress, lower inflammation, and improve overall brain health, antioxidants are crucial for preserving cognitive function and delaying the onset of AD.

Following the principles of the Mediterranean diet may offer a holistic approach to Alzheimer's disease prevention, emphasizing the importance of dietary modifications in improving cognitive performance and impeding.

Understanding of Alzheimer's Pathophysiology

Amyloid Beta (Aβ) plaques and neurofibrillary tangles: An buildup of Aβ plaque and hyper phosphorylated tau protein that results in neuronal dysfunction and cell death. Oxidative Stress: Oxidative stress is defined as an increase in the production of reactive oxygen species (ROS), which damages cells. Long-term astrocyte and microglia activation that causes neurodegeneration is known as neuro inflammation.

Impaired Neurotransmission: This occurs when the glutamate and cholinergic neurotransmitter networks are disrupted.

Potential Neuroprotective Mechanisms:

a. Anti-Amyloid Strategies:

Targeting enzymes involved in the formation of Aβ, β-Secretase (BACE) Inhibitors are one type of anti-amyloid strategy. Immunotherapy: Boosting immune function to eliminate Aβ plaques.

b. Anti-Tau Therapies:

Inhibitors of Tau Kinase: Preventing the enzymes that cause hyper phosphorylation of tau. Tau Aggregation Inhibitors: Stopping neurofibrillary tangles from forming.

c. Blends of Antioxidants:

Fruits, vegetables, and green tea all include polyphenols, which are compounds with antioxidant qualities.

d. Vitamins C and E:

They lower oxidative stress and scavenge free radicals.

Round Anti-inflammatory Agents:

Neuro inflammation is modulated by nonsteroidal anti-inflammatory drugs (NSAIDs).

Cannabinoids: lowering inflammation and controlling immunological responses.

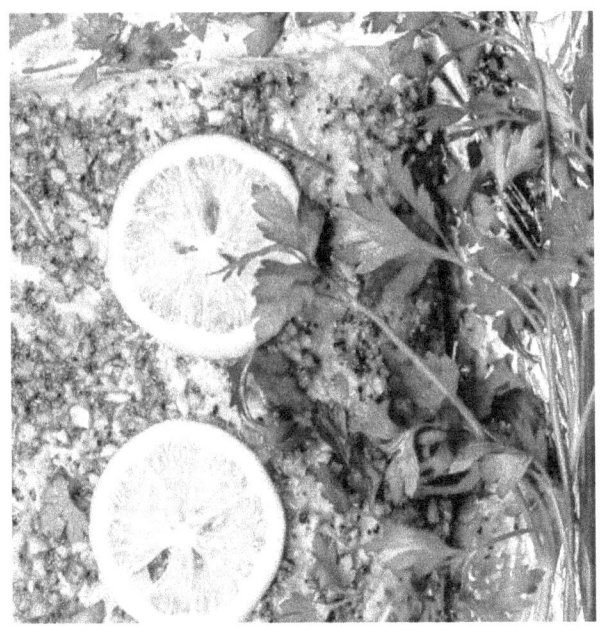

Emerging Neuroprotective Compounds and Therapies:

a. Neurotrophic factors: Encouraging synaptic plasticity and neuronal survival.

b. Metabolic modulators: Improving energy metabolism and mitochondrial performance.

c. Epigenetic Alterers: Controlling the expression of genes linked to neurodegeneration.

d. Stem Cell Therapy: Fostering regeneration and repairing damaged neural circuitry.

Lifestyle Interventions for Neuroprotection:

a. Exercise: Improving cognitive function and reducing the risk of AD.

b. Engaging in mentally taxing activities stimulates the brain.

c. Healthy Diet: A healthy diet consists of a well-balanced food that is rich in antioxidants and omega-3 fatty acids.

d. Sufficient Sleep: Sleep is essential for brain function and memory consolidation.

Challenges and Future Directions:

Transitioning from preclinical research to clinical application: Overcoming translational hurdles. Multimodal Approaches: Blending several neuroprotective methods to produce supplementary effects. The practice of creating interventions based on a patient's particular genetic and environmental composition is known as personalized medicine.

As the prevalence of Alzheimer's disease increases worldwide, there is an increasing demand for efficient neuroprotective techniques. Neurodegeneration may be slowed by a wide range of drugs and treatments, but numerous challenges must be solved before these findings may be used in therapeutic settings.

Long-term research, combined with creative thinking and collaborative efforts, is essential to revealing potential neuroprotective advantages against Alzheimer's and improving the quality of life for those affected by the illness.

Incorporating Antioxidant-Rich Foods into Daily Diet

Antioxidants are substances that neutralize free radicals, which are unstable atoms that can harm cells, ageing, and diseases like cancer, cardiovascular disease, and cognitive loss. By scavenging free radicals, antioxidants help protect cells from oxidative damage, reducing the risk of chronic disorders and extending life.

Types of Antioxidants:

Vitamin C: Found in abundance in bell peppers, broccoli, citrus fruits, strawberries, kiwis, and other foods, vitamin C supports the production of collagen and fortifies the immune system.

Vitamin E: Vitamin E protects cell membranes from oxidative damage and is present in avocados, almonds, seeds, spinach, and other plant foods. It also helps to maintain healthy skin.

Beta-carotene: Spinach, kale, carrots, and sweet potatoes are rich sources of beta-carotene, which aids in the body's production of vitamin A, which is necessary for a strong immune system and eyesight.

Selenium: This mineral maintains the functioning of the thyroid and immune system by acting as a cofactor for antioxidant enzymes. It can be found in whole grains, seafood, poultry, and Brazil nuts.

Flavonoids: Found in tea, dark chocolate, berries, and citrus fruits, flavonoids have anti-inflammatory and antioxidant qualities that support heart health and brain function.

Incorporating Antioxidant-Rich Foods into Your Daily Diet:

Start Your Day with Berries: Add a handful of blueberries, strawberries, or raspberries to your breakfast cereal, yogurt, or smoothie for a potent antioxidant boost.

Snack on Nuts and Seeds: For an easy, high-antioxidant snack, keep a supply of almonds, walnuts, pumpkin seeds, or sunflower seeds on hand.

Emphasize Leafy Greens: To boost your intake of antioxidants and vital nutrients, add spinach, kale, Swiss chard, or collard greens to salads, soups, stir-fries, or smoothies.

Select Vibrant Vegetables: Choose a rainbow of veggies, such as tomatoes, bell peppers, carrots, and sweet potatoes, to increase the variety in your antioxidant intake and to improve the appearance of your food.

Savor Herbal Teas: To stay hydrated and benefit from plant-based antioxidants, sip antioxidant-rich herbal teas like chamomile, green tea, or rooibos throughout the day.

Enjoy Dark Chocolate: Give yourself a square of dark chocolate that has at least 70% cocoa content to sate your sweet tooth and reap the advantages of flavonoids, which are antioxidants.

Add Flavor to Your Meals: Spices and herbs high in antioxidants, such as cloves, cinnamon, ginger, turmeric, and oregano, can enhance the flavor and nutritional value of your cuisine.

In conclusion, you may strengthen your body's defensive mechanisms against oxidative stress and chronic diseases while also providing your body with necessary nutrients by including foods high in antioxidants in your regular diet. To live a lively and fulfilling life, embrace a wide variety of colorful fruits, vegetables, nuts, seeds, and spices. As you go out on a path towards health and vitality, let your plate serve as a painting.

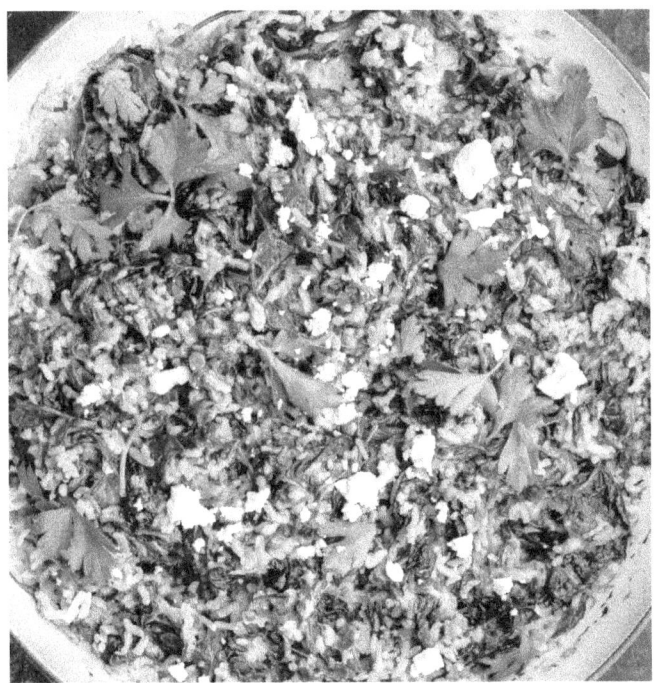

CHAPTER 7: GUT MICROBIOTA AND COGNITIVE HEALTH

Gut Microbiota and Alzheimer's Disease:

The varied ecology of bacteria known as the gut microbiota, which inhabits the gastrointestinal tract, is essential for immunological control, metabolism, and neurobehavioral processes, among other physiological activities.

New research points to the gut-brain axis as a bidirectional communication pathway where changes in the makeup of the gut bacteria can affect brain function and vice versa. Unbalances in the gut microbial populations, or dysbiosis, have been linked to a number of neurological conditions, including Alzheimer's disease.

Influence of Diet on Gut Microbiota Composition:

Food habits have a big impact on the variety and makeup of gut bacteria. Some food ingredients, like fiber, prebiotics, and polyphenols, encourage the growth of good bacteria, whereas other ingredients, like sugar and saturated fats, can negatively impact microbial communities.

Rich in fruits, vegetables, and whole grains, high-fiber diets encourage the growth of good bacteria like Lactobacilli and Bifidobacteria, which support gut health and may have neuroprotective properties.

Diets high in processed foods and saturated fats, on the other hand, have been linked to dysbiosis, heightened vulnerability to neuro inflammation, and cognitive impairment.

Role of Gut Microbiota in Neuro inflammation and Alzheimer's Pathology:

Alzheimer's disease pathogenesis is characterized by persistent inflammation and dysregulated immunological responses.
The blood-brain barrier's integrity may be compromised by gut dysbiosis, which can lead to systemic inflammation and make it easier for neurotoxic chemicals to enter the brain.

Short-chain fatty acids (SCFAs) and lipopolysaccharides (LPS), two metabolites made by gut microorganisms, have the ability to alter neuro inflammatory pathways and affect the aggregation of tau and amyloid-beta proteins, which are the two main markers of Alzheimer's disease.

Dietary Interventions for Alzheimer's Prevention and Management:

Dietary therapies with specific targets to alter the composition of the gut microbiota have potential for managing and preventing Alzheimer's disease.

A diet high in fruits, vegetables, whole grains, seafood, and healthy fats, known as the Mediterranean diet, has been linked to a lower risk of Alzheimer's disease and cognitive decline.

Certain dietary elements, including probiotics, polyphenols, and omega-3 fatty acids, have been shown to have neuroprotective qualities and to help reduce oxidative stress and neuro inflammation.

Personalized nutrition strategies based on unique gut microbiota profiles have the potential to improve therapeutic results and boost the effectiveness of dietary therapies for Alzheimer's patients.

Future Directions and Clinical Implications:

To fully understand the intricate relationships between gut microbiota, nutrition, and the pathophysiology of Alzheimer's disease, more investigation is necessary. To prove causation and provide evidence for evidence-based dietary recommendations, longitudinal studies examining the impact of dietary interventions on gut microbiota dynamics and cognitive outcomes are required.

The incorporation of dietary adjustments and medicines targeting the gut microbiota into comprehensive approaches to managing Alzheimer's disease has the potential to slow down the illness's course and enhance patient outcomes.

Comprehending the complex relationship among nutrition, gut microbiota, and Alzheimer's disease offers new perspectives on both preventive and treatment measures for this crippling neurodegenerative condition.

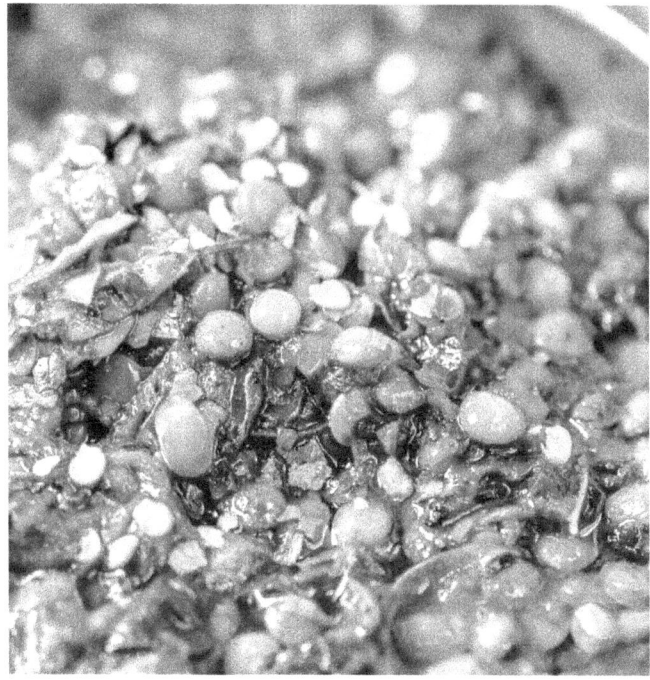

Diversity of Gut Microbiota and the Mediterranean Diet

Gut Microbiota Diversity and Brain Health: The billions of microorganisms that live in the gastrointestinal tract are known as the gut microbiota, and they are essential for immune system function, digestion, and nutrient absorption. The gut-brain axis is a two-way communication pathway that facilitates communication between the gut and the brain. According to emerging studies, the diversity and composition of gut bacteria may have an impact on brain health.

Alzheimer's Disease and Gut Microbiota:

Alzheimer's disease is a neurological condition that worsens with time and is marked by behavioral abnormalities, memory loss, and cognitive impairment. Although the precise etiology of Alzheimer's disease is still unknown, mounting data indicates that changes in the variety and composition of gut microbes—a condition known as gut microbiota dysbiosis—may have a role in the onset and progression of the illness.

The Role of the Mediterranean Diet in Gut Microbiota Diversity:

Following the Mediterranean diet is linked to a more varied and well-balanced makeup of the gut microbiota, according to several studies. The Mediterranean diet's high fiber and plant-based food intake encourages the growth of lactobacilli and Bifidobacteria, two types of good bacteria, while lowering the number of dangerous microorganisms.

Consuming olive oil, which is high in polyphenols and monounsaturated fats, has also been demonstrated to have anti-inflammatory and antioxidant qualities, which may help to maintain gut health.

Implications for Alzheimer's Disease Prevention:

Following the Mediterranean diet may help maintain a diversified and healthy gut microbiota, which may have important implications for preventing Alzheimer's disease. The growth of tau tangles, amyloid-beta plaques, and neuro inflammation—all of which are characteristic signs of Alzheimer's disease—may be lessened by maintaining a healthy gut flora, according to research.

Implications for Alzheimer's Disease Prevention and Treatment

1. Early Detection and Diagnosis

Effective management and intervention of Alzheimer's disease depend heavily on early detection. Technological developments in neuroimaging, biomarker research, and genetic testing have made it possible to diagnose patients more quickly and accurately, which has accelerated their access to support services and the right care. Early diagnosis also makes it easier to put targeted interventions and lifestyle changes into practice that delay the progression of the condition.

2. Lifestyle Modifications

There is mounting evidence that suggests certain lifestyle choices may impact one's risk of Alzheimer's disease. A healthy lifestyle that includes cognitive stimulation, frequent exercise, a diet rich in fruits, vegetables, and omega-3 fatty acids, enough sleep, and physical activity may help lower the risk of dementia and cognitive decline. Furthermore, controlling cardiovascular risk factors like diabetes, obesity, smoking, and hypertension can improve general brain health and possibly reduce the incidence of Alzheimer's disease.

3. Pharmacological Interventions

Although there isn't a cure for Alzheimer's disease at the moment, pharmaceutical therapies try to lessen symptoms and enhance the lives of those who have the illness. Memantine and cholinesterase inhibitors are two often given drugs that address neurotransmitter imbalances in the brain to assist treat behavioral and cognitive problems. These medications, however, have negligible side effects and do not stop the underlying disease from progressing.

4. Disease-Modifying Therapies

One of the main areas of scientific investigation has been the development of disease-modifying treatments for Alzheimer's disease. The underlying pathogenic processes, such as the buildup of tau protein tangles and amyloid-beta plaques in the brain, are the focus of these treatments.

Clinical trials are now being conducted to investigate a number of potential therapies, such as beta-secretase inhibitors, tau aggregation inhibitors, and monoclonal antibodies. The development of effective medicines to reduce disease progression is still elusive, despite some encouraging outcomes being reported.

5. Personalized Medicine

In Alzheimer's research, the idea of personalized medicine is gaining support as it acknowledges the disease's variability and the significance of tailored methods to prevention and therapy. The identification of particular risk factors and disease subtypes is made possible by genetic profiling, biomarker analysis, and neuroimaging approaches.

This opens the door to customized therapies that cater to the individual needs of every patient. In the fight against Alzheimer's disease, precision medicine offers the potential to improve patient care and treatment outcomes.

6. Non-Pharmacological Interventions

Non-pharmacological interventions are essential for treating the symptoms of Alzheimer's disease and improving quality of life in addition to pharmaceutical treatments. These therapies cover a broad spectrum of techniques, such as psychotherapy, music therapy, art therapy, cognitive rehabilitation, and recollection therapy. In addition, community-based services and caregiver support programs are critical to providing comprehensive care and support for people with Alzheimer's disease and their families.

7. Ethical and Societal Implications

It is critical to discuss the ethical and societal ramifications of Alzheimer's disease prevention and therapy as research advances and new therapies become available. Careful thought must be given to issues including informed consent, genetic testing, end-of-life decision-making, healthcare inequities, and access to care in order to guarantee fair and humane treatment for all those impacted by the illness. In addition, creating dementia-friendly communities, lowering stigma, and increasing knowledge are crucial for promoting compassion and understanding for those with Alzheimer's disease.

Even though our understanding of the condition has advanced significantly, there is still more to be done to create supportive networks and effective treatments that will improve the prognosis and quality of life for those who have Alzheimer's disease.

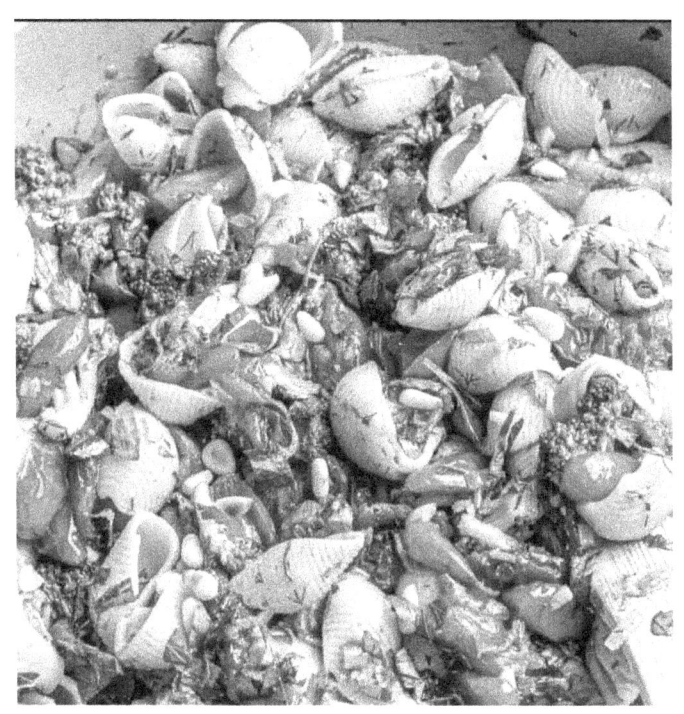

CHAPTER 8:
MEAL PLANNING AND RECIPES

Practical Tips for Adopting Mediterranean Diet

This diet plan has a strong emphasis on plant-based foods, healthy fats, and moderation in the consumption of fish and poultry. It is modeled after the typical eating patterns of Mediterranean Sea coast countries. Here are some doable suggestions for adopting a Mediterranean diet to help lessen the impact of Alzheimer's disease.

Emphasize Plant-Based Foods:

Arrange a bright platter of fruits and vegetables that are high in vitamins, minerals, and antioxidants.

Try to obtain at least five servings of fruits and vegetables each day, such as cruciferous vegetables like broccoli and cauliflower, leafy greens, berries, and tomatoes. For long-lasting energy and fiber, include whole grains like quinoa, brown rice, whole wheat bread, and oats in your meals.

Choose Healthy Fats:

Choose olive oil as your main fat source and use it for dips, salad dressings, and cooking. Particularly abundant in anti-inflammatory and antioxidant substances is extra virgin olive oil.

Add heart-healthy fats and vital nutrients to your diet by include nuts and seeds like flaxseeds, chia seeds, walnuts, and almonds.

Reduce your intake of processed foods, fried foods, and fatty meats that include saturated and trans fats, as these can worsen inflammation and lead to cognitive loss.

Prioritize Fish and Lean Protein:

Omega-3 fatty acids are essential for brain health and may lower the incidence of Alzheimer's disease. Eat fatty fish, such as salmon, sardines, and mackerel, at least twice a week to reap their benefits.

To promote muscular health and general well-being, include lean protein sources like chicken, eggs, lentils, and tofu in your meals.
When it comes to red meat, consider lean cuts like tenderloin or sirloin or limit your intake and consume smaller portions.

Include Dairy in Moderation:

For sources of calcium and protein, choose for dairy products like yogurt, cheese, and milk that are low in fat or fat free. Choose calcium-enriched dairy-free yogurt and

cheese, as well as fortified soy or almond milk, if you'd rather go plant-based.
Reduce your consumption of high-fat dairy products like whole milk and full-fat cheeses because consuming too much saturated fat raises your risk of cognitive decline.

Enjoy Herbs and Spices:

Use herbs and spices to add flavor to your food rather than adding too much salt or sugar to make it taste better without sacrificing health.
Try experimenting with Mediterranean herbs to give your cooking more flavor and aroma, such as basil, oregano, thyme, and rosemary.
Add spices like ginger, cinnamon, and turmeric, which have anti-inflammatory qualities and may improve cognitive function.

Stay Hydrated:

Throughout the day, sip on lots of water to stay hydrated and promote healthy brain function. Aim for 8 to 10 glasses of water a day, more or less depending on your needs and degree of activity.
Avoid sugar-filled drinks like soda and fruit juices and instead choose herbal teas, water, or water that has been infused with fresh fruit and herbs for flavor.

Practice Mindful Eating:

To improve enjoyment and aid in digestion, take your time and enjoy every bite, paying attention to flavors, textures, and feelings.

Stay away from screens and multitasking when you eat so that you can give your whole attention to the process of fueling your body and mind.

Pay attention to your body's signals of hunger and fullness, and stop eating when you're satisfied but not too full.

Sample Meal Plans for Different Dietary Preferences

This guide will walk you through sample meal plans that may be customized to fit a variety of dietary needs and enhance the brain health and wellbeing of people with Alzheimer's disease.

Mediterranean Diet Meal Plan:

The benefits of the Mediterranean diet on the brain are widely recognized, and it has been associated with a lower risk of cognitive decline. This menu consists of:

Breakfast: Greek yogurt, berries, and almonds, along with whole-grain toast topped with olive oil, is what I have for breakfast.
Lunch: Consists of quinoa, roasted veggies, and grilled salmon.
Snack: Carrot sticks with hummus.
Dinner: Whole-grain pita bread, Greek salad, and chicken souvlaki.
Dessert: A fresh fruit salad dressed with honey.

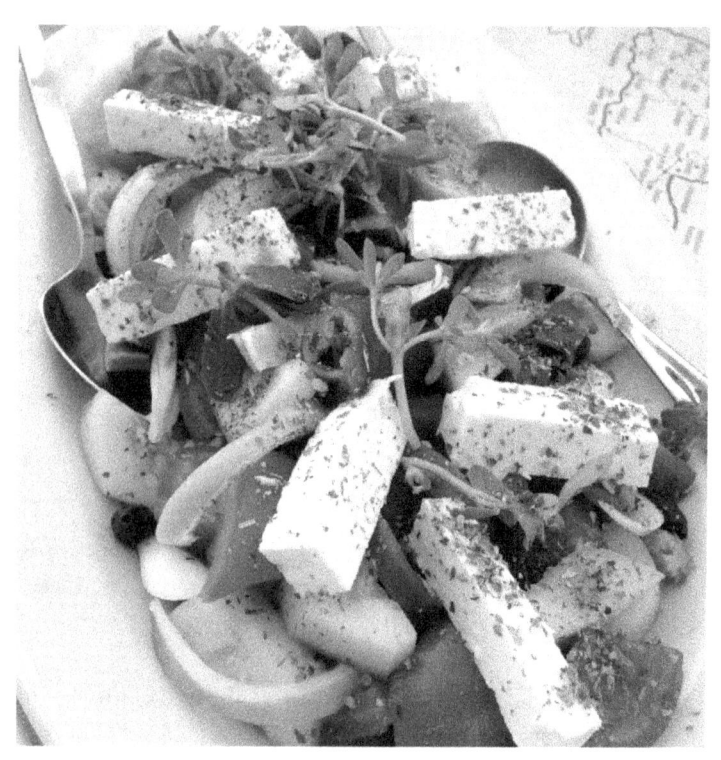

DASH Diet Meal Plan:

The Dietary Approaches to Stop Hypertension (DASH) diet is a good way to manage Alzheimer's symptoms since it places an emphasis on whole grains, fruits, vegetables, lean proteins, and low-fat dairy products. This is an example of a menu:
Breakfast: Consists of oatmeal with almonds and sliced banana on top.
Lunch: consists of a wrap with turkey and avocado and a side salad.
Snack: Peach slices paired with Greek yogurt.
Dinner: Steamed broccoli and baked chicken breast paired with quinoa for dinner.
Dissert: Apples baked with cinnamon for dessert.

Plant-Based Diet Meal Plan:

For those suffering from Alzheimer's disease, a plant-based diet high in fruits, vegetables, legumes, nuts, and seeds can offer enough nutrition and reduce inflammation. This is an example of a menu:
Breast: Smoothie for breakfast consisting of spinach, banana, almond milk, and chia seeds.
Lunch: Would include a side of whole-grain bread and a soup of lentils and vegetables.
Snack: Dried fruit and mixed nuts.
Dinner: is brown rice and stir-fried tofu with mixed vegetables.
Dessert: Pudding made with chia seeds and delicious berries.

Low-Carb/Ketogenic Diet Meal Plan:

According to some research, a low-carb or ketogenic diet may help people with Alzheimer's disease by giving their brains other source of energy. This is an example of a menu:
Breast: Avocado and spinach scrambled eggs for breakfast.
Lunch: would be a low-carb Caesar salad with grilled chicken.
Snacks: Cheese with cucumber slices for a snack.
Dinner: is a side salad dressed with olive oil and baked salmon served with asparagus.
Dessert: Whipped cream and sugar-free jello.

Developing a healthy diet based on personal tastes is essential for Alzheimer's disease management. It doesn't matter if you're on a plant-based, low-carb/ketogenic, DASH, or Mediterranean diet—the important thing is to focus on full, nutrient-dense meals and limit processed and added sugars.

To further customize meal plans and provide the best possible nutrition for those with Alzheimer's disease, speak with a medical professional or registered dietitian.
Simple and Tasty Recipes with Mediterranean Flavors

A few quick and delectable Mediterranean-inspired meals that are full of nutrients that may help Alzheimer's sufferers.

Mediterranean Chickpea Salad:

Ingredients:

Legumes, rinsed and drained, in one can
One each of cucumber and tomato slices
1/4 cup of red onion, thinly sliced
quarter cup freshly chopped parsley
A quarter cup of feta cheese in crumbles
Two teaspoons of finely chopped olive oil
One teaspoon of lemon juice
To taste, add more salt and pepper.

Guidelines:

Chickpeas, cucumber, tomato, red onion, and parsley should all be combined in a big bowl.

In a small bowl, whisk together the olive oil, lemon juice, salt, and pepper.

Pour the dressing over the salad and toss to coat.

Before serving, sprinkle some feta cheese on top.

Grilled Mediterranean Chicken:

Ingredients:

Four skinless, boneless chicken breasts
Two teaspoons of pure olive oil and two sliced garlic cloves
One tablespoon of oregano, dried
One tsp of thyme, dried

Half a teaspoon of rosemary, dried
To taste, add more salt and pepper.

Guidelines:

Combine the olive oil, garlic, thyme, rosemary, oregano, and salt & pepper in a small bowl.

The chicken breasts should be rubbed with the mixture and let to marinade for at least half an hour.

Turn the grill up to medium-high and cook the chicken for 6 to 8 minutes on each side, or until it's thoroughly done. For a full supper, serve with whole grain couscous and a side of Greek salad.

Roasted Vegetables in the Mediterranean:

Ingredients:

Four skinless, boneless chicken breasts
Two teaspoons of pure olive oil and two sliced garlic cloves
One tablespoon of oregano, dried
One tsp of thyme, dried
Half a teaspoon of rosemary, dried
To taste, add more salt and pepper.

Guidelines:
Turn the oven on to 400°F, or 200°C. Combine all the vegetables in a big bowl with the olive oil, oregano, garlic, salt, and pepper.

Arrange the veggies on a baking pan so they are in a single layer.

Roast the vegetables for 25 to 30 minutes in a preheated oven, or until they are soft and have a hint of caramelization.

For a heartier meal, serve over cooked quinoa or as a side dish.

Mediterranean Yogurt Parfait:

Ingredients:

One cup of Greek yogurt
Half a cup of mixed berries, including blueberries, raspberries, and strawberries
1/4 cup finely chopped walnuts or almonds
Just one tablespoon of honey

Guidelines:

Toss together Greek yogurt, sliced almonds, and mixed berries in a glass or dish; drizzle with honey to sweeten even more.

This can be a healthy breakfast choice or a light dessert.

Including meals with a Mediterranean flair in the diet can have several health advantages, such as promoting brain function and possibly lowering the chance of cognitive decline brought on by Alzheimer's disease.

These simple and tasty dishes provide a tasty method to enhance general well-being while also nourishing the body and mind. We can actively support mental health and lead bright, satisfying lives by embracing the flavors of the Mediterranean diet.

CHAPTER 9:
LIFESTYLE FACTORS AND ALZHEIMER'S PREVENTION

Beyond Diet: Importance of Physical Activity

The significance of lifestyle factors, such as nutrition and exercise, in determining the risk and course of Alzheimer's disease has come to the attention of scientists more and more in recent years.

Physical activity is one of these elements that stands out as being very effective in maintaining resilience against cognitive decline and brain health. Regular exercise has been repeatedly demonstrated to help reduce the risk of Alzheimer's disease and decrease the disease's progression in those who already have it.

Advantages of Exercise for Alzheimer's Patients:

Brain Health: Engaging in physical activity causes the brain to release chemicals that encourage the development of new brain cells and the connections that connect them. This neuroplasticity process may possibly counteract the consequences of brain alterations associated with

Alzheimer's disease. It aids in the maintenance of cognitive function.

Decreased Inflammation: Alzheimer's disease is thought to be significantly influenced by chronic inflammation. Frequent exercise has been demonstrated to lower inflammation in the brain as well as other parts of the body, which may help prevent brain injury and cognitive deterioration.

Better Blood Flow: Exercise improves blood flow, which lowers the risk of atherosclerosis and high blood pressure while also improving cardiovascular health. Toxin removal, oxygen and nutrition delivery, and brain function all depend on the brain receiving enough blood flow.

Enhanced Emotion and Well-Being: Alzheimer's disease has a negative impact on emotional and psychological well-being in addition to its effects on cognitive performance. Exercise has been demonstrated to increase mood, lower stress and anxiety, and enhance overall quality of life for both caregivers and those with Alzheimer's disease.

Including Physical Activity in Daily Life: Although there is little doubt about the health benefits of physical activity for Alzheimer's patients, many people may find it difficult to start and stick to an exercise program, particularly when dealing with physical and mental difficulties.

I Am Even Little Adjustments Can Have an Impact:

Start Slowly: Take it easy and start with fun hobbies like dancing, strolling, or gardening. As tolerated, progressively increase the time and intensity.

Make it Social: To maintain accountability and motivation, work out with friends, family, or in a group. Emotional support and cognitive stimulation are further benefits of social connection.

Adjust as Necessary: Adapt activities to each person's capabilities and preferences. Think about utilizing assistive technology or getting advice from a fitness expert or physical therapist.

Remain Consistent: Try to get moving on a regular basis, preferably with a combination of strength, flexibility, and cardio workouts. To experience the long-term advantages for brain health, consistency is essential.

Stress Management and Adequate Sleep

The Impact of Stress on Brain Health:

Prolonged stress can cause inflammation, oxidative stress, and dysregulation of different neurotransmitter systems, all of which can have negative consequences on the brain. Long-term exposure to stress hormones like cortisol can alter the structure of important brain regions involved in memory and cognition, like the prefrontal cortex and hippocampus, and disrupt neuronal communication. Furthermore, a higher chance of developing AD pathology, such as the buildup of tau tangles and beta-amyloid plaques, has been connected to persistent stress.

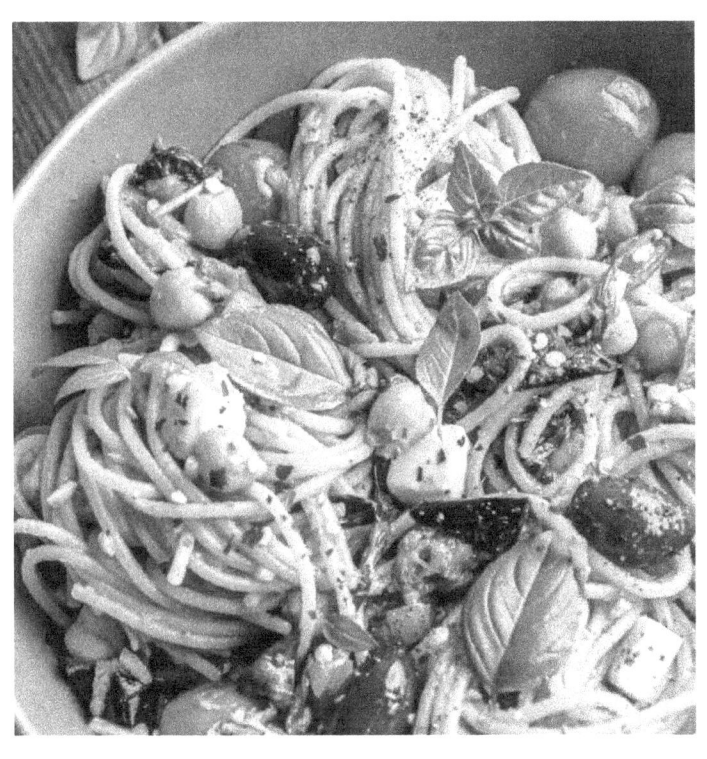

105 | MEDITTERRANEAN DIET FOR ALZHEIMERS DISEASE

Strategies for Stress Management:

It takes effective stress management to protect the brain and lower the risk of Alzheimer's. Daily implementation of stress-reduction practices can help lessen the negative physiological and psychological impacts of stress. These could include practicing progressive muscular relaxation, yoga, deep breathing techniques, mindfulness meditation, and spending time in nature. Engaging in joyful and fulfilling hobbies and building a supportive social network are further strategies to mitigate the damaging effects of stress on the brain.

The Role of Sleep in Brain Health:

Sleep is necessary for brain detoxification, memory consolidation, and cognitive function. The brain eliminates toxins when we sleep, one of which is beta-amyloid, which has been linked to the onset of Alzheimer's disease. These vital processes are disrupted by persistent sleep deprivation or disruptions, which raises the risk of neurodegeneration and cognitive decline. A higher chance of developing AD and a higher deposition of beta-amyloid plaques have been linked to poor sleep quality.

Promoting Healthy Sleep Habits:

Prioritizing good sleep hygiene is paramount for maintaining optimal brain health and reducing the risk of Alzheimer's disease. Establishing a regular sleep schedule, creating a restful sleep environment, and avoiding stimulants like caffeine and electronic devices before bedtime can improve sleep quality.

Relaxation techniques, such as guided imagery or bedtime yoga, can help calm the mind and facilitate sleep onset. Additionally, seeking treatment for sleep disorders like insomnia or sleep apnea is crucial for optimizing sleep and minimizing Alzheimer's risk.

The growing body of research on Alzheimer's disease is making it more and more clear that lifestyle choices like stress reduction and getting enough sleep are critical for maintaining brain function and preventing the illness. People might potentially lower their risk of Alzheimer's disease and improve their overall quality of life by proactively reducing stress and prioritizing appropriate sleep habits.

Promoting brain resilience and maintaining cognitive function across the lifetime requires adopting a holistic approach to well-being that takes into account both physical and mental health.

Social Engagement and Mental Stimulation

Participating in significant conversations and activities inside one's social network is referred to as social engagement. Keeping up social ties is crucial for people with Alzheimer's disease for a number of reasons:

Cognitive Stimulation: Social interaction improves memory, focus, and problem-solving abilities, among other cognitive abilities. Participating in social activities, games, and conversations can assist maintain cognitive function and train the brain.

Emotional Well-Being: Engaging in social contacts can help reduce feelings of depression and loneliness that are frequently linked to Alzheimer's disease. These connections also offer emotional support and a sense of belonging. Participating in social events and spending time with loved ones can improve one's mood and general quality of life.

Stimulation of Neural Pathways: Social interaction stimulates the brain's neural pathways, allowing brain cells to communicate with one another and possibly delaying the onset of cognitive decline. Frequent social contact may protect brain health and postpone the development of more serious symptoms.

Strategies for Enhancing Social Engagement:

Encourage involvement in community programs: A lot of places provide recreational opportunities, memory cafes, and support groups especially for people with Alzheimer's disease and their carriers.

Foster meaningful connections: Encourage opportunities to participate in common interests and hobbies, as well as family and friend visits, to cultivate deep and lasting relationships.

Make use of technology: Social media and video calls are examples of virtual communication platforms that can help you stay in touch with loved ones who live far away.

The Importance of Mental Stimulation:

Mental stimulation is just as important for treating Alzheimer's disease as social interaction. Activities that test and exercise the brain, fostering neuronal plasticity and cognitive performance, are referred to as mental stimulation. Among the main advantages of mental stimulation are:

Cognitive Reserve: The capacity of the brain to tolerate damage and continue to operate normally in spite of age-related changes or neurological diseases is known as cognitive reserve, and it is increased by mentally demanding activities. Higher cognitive reserve people might have less symptoms and a slower rate of illness progression.

Neuroplasticity: The brain's capacity to remodel and create new neural connections in response to experience and learning is facilitated by mental stimulation. Through consistent mental challenges like reading, puzzles, and acquiring new abilities, people can improve their cognitive flexibility and adaptability.

Better Brain Health: Research has linked regular mental stimulation to a lower risk of cognitive decline and a higher state of brain health. Those who maintain an active and engaged brain may benefit from improved memory, focus, and general cognitive function.

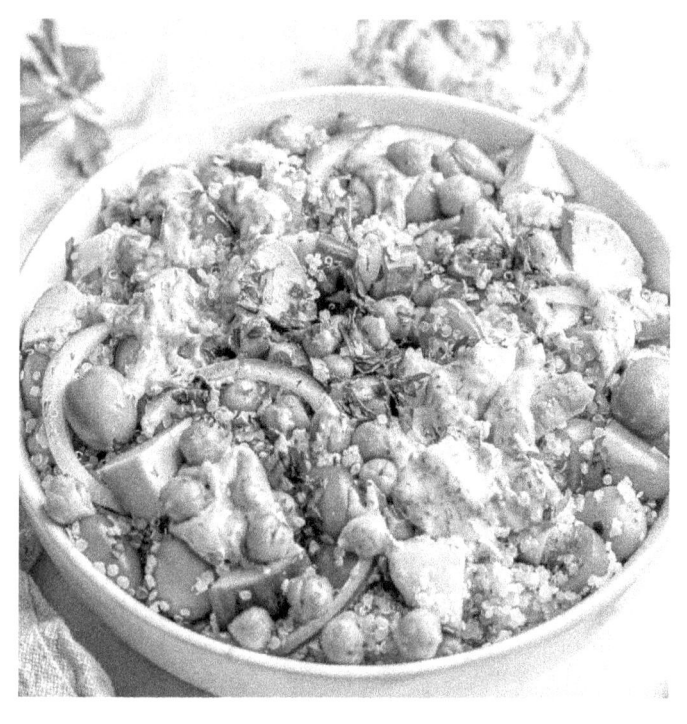

Strategies for Promoting Mental Stimulation:

Take part in cognitive exercises: Promote the completion of mental exercises like Sudoku, crossword puzzles, and memory games.

Accept lifelong education: Adopt interests, pastimes, and educational endeavors that enhance mental capacity and foster intellectual development.

Ensure a setting that is stimulating: Provide a space that is suited for cerebral stimulation by providing art, music, books, and other stimulating activities.

A holistic approach to managing Alzheimer's disease must include social engagement and mental stimulation. Through meaningful social connections and mentally stimulating activities, people with Alzheimer's can improve their emotional and cognitive functioning, potentially delaying the disease's progression.

Communities, caregivers, and healthcare professionals are essential in supporting and promoting social engagement and mental stimulation for those living with Alzheimer's disease, ultimately improving their quality of life and well-being.

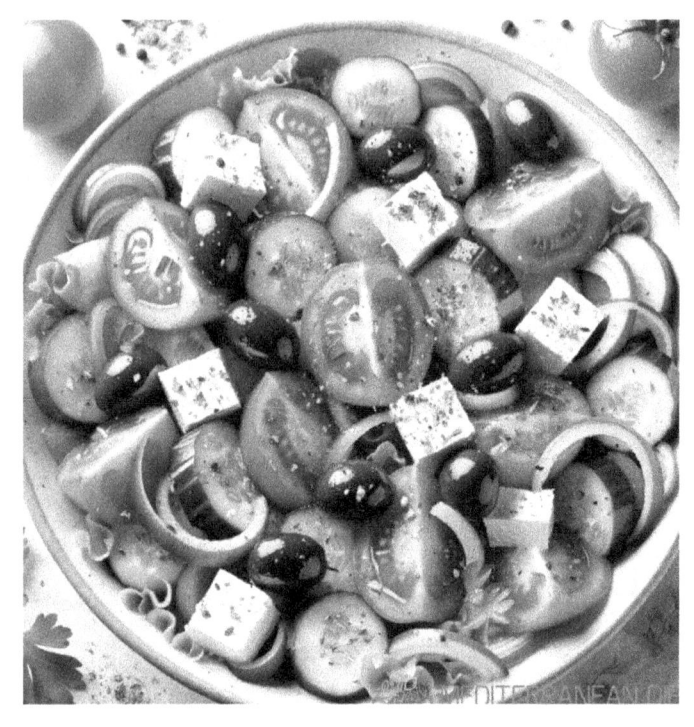

CHAPTER 10:
IMPLEMENTING THE MEDITERRANEAN DIET FOR ALZHEIMER'S PREVENTION

Steps to Start Incorporating Mediterranean Diet

Step 1: Understand the Mediterranean Diet

An abundance of plant-based foods, including fruits, vegetables, legumes, and whole grains, is a hallmark of the Mediterranean diet. Along with minimal intake of red meat, it also entails moderate eating of fish, poultry, and dairy items. In this diet, healthy fats—especially those found in nuts, seeds, and olive oil—are essential. Gaining an understanding of the fundamentals of the Mediterranean diet is the first step towards implementing it into your regular eating routine.

Step 2: Stock Up on Mediterranean Staples

Start by filling your fridge and pantry with essential items so you can start implementing the Mediterranean diet into your daily routine. Among them are:
Extra virgin olive oil for salad dressing and cooking.
entire grains such as whole wheat pasta, quinoa, and brown rice.
Lots of fresh produce, with an emphasis on a range of hues and varieties.
Lentils, fish, chicken, and eggs are examples of lean proteins.
Nuts and seeds to add to meals or as a snack.
Spices and herbs can be used in place of salt to flavor food.

Step 3: Plan Balanced Meals

Accept the moderation, diversity, and balance of the Mediterranean meal planning philosophy. Try to load up on these:
Vegetables: Whether they are the main course, a salad, or a side dish, add a rainbow of colors to every meal.
Fruits: Eat fresh fruits for breakfast or as a side dish with savory foods. You may also enjoy them as snacks or desserts.
Whole grains: To boost satiety and enhance fiber consumption, choose for whole grain options like bread, pasta, and rice.
Lean proteins: For protein, iron, and other vital elements, include fish, poultry, eggs, and lentils in your diet.
Healthy fats: Your main source of fat should be olive oil.

You may also add nuts, seeds, and avocado to salads, yoghurt, and snacks.

Step 4: Be Mindful of Portions

The Mediterranean diet promotes diversity in food, but in order to keep a healthy weight and avoid overindulging, portion control is crucial. Observe portion sizes and pay attention to your body's signals of hunger and fullness. Consuming less calories can be achieved by eating mindfully, slowly, and only quitting when you're full.

Step 5: Stay Hydrated and Stay Active

Consuming food in the Mediterranean manner, drinking enough of water, and exercising frequently are all essential elements of a healthy lifestyle. Throughout the day, sip on lots of water, avoid sugar-filled drinks, and indulge in flavorful herbal teas or infused water. Every day of the week, try to get in at least 30 minutes of moderate-intensity activity. You can mix in enjoyable exercises like dancing, swimming, or walking.

Step 6: Seek Professional Guidance and Support

See a qualified dietician or other healthcare professional if you're not sure where to begin or have specific health concerns. They may offer you customized advice based on your requirements and support you in overcoming any obstacles you may come across. Joining support groups or taking Mediterranean-inspired cooking classes can also offer inspiration, drive, and a feeling of community.

Including a Mediterranean diet in your daily routine is a proactive way to support cognitive function and lower your risk of Alzheimer's. You may fuel your body and mind for long-term well-being by appreciating balance and moderation, giving priority to nutrient-dense foods, and maintaining an active lifestyle. Start small, try out different products and dishes, and acknowledge and appreciate your progress toward a healthy you.

Overcoming Challenges and Barriers

People may need more help with everyday tasks as their illness worsens, which could eventually necessitate full-time care.

Problems that People with Alzheimer's Disease Face:

Memory Loss and Cognitive Decline: Two of the main signs of Alzheimer's disease are forgetfulness and confusion, which make it difficult for sufferers to recall crucial details like names, appointments, and recent occurrences. Frustration, anxiety, and a decline in self-confidence might result from this.

Communication Problems: Alzheimer's disease can impede linguistic abilities, making it challenging for sufferers to explain themselves or comprehend others. Both the Alzheimer's patient and their carriers may experience feelings of frustration and loneliness as a result of this communication failure.

Daily Living Challenges: As the illness worsens, people may find it difficult to carry out daily activities including dressing, eating, and taking a shower. It can be upsetting to lose independence, and caregivers may need to provide a lot of support.

Behavioral and Psychological Symptoms: Agitation, depression, hallucinations, and agitation are just a few of the behavioral and psychological symptoms that Alzheimer's disease can cause. It can be difficult to manage these symptoms, and doing so frequently calls for a multimodal strategy that includes medication, behavioral treatments, and environment changes.

Caregiver Burden: Providing medical, psychological, and financial support to a loved one suffering from Alzheimer's disease can be taxing. High levels of stress, burnout, and social isolation may be experienced by caregivers, which can negatively affect their own health and wellbeing.

Methods for Getting Through Obstacles and Difficulties:

Education and Assistance: Acquiring knowledge about the course of Alzheimer's disease and mastering efficient caregiving techniques will enable patients and their carriers to more effectively handle the difficulties brought on by the illness. Important resources and emotional support can be obtained by joining support groups, going to educational programs, and consulting medical professionals.

Simplification and Adaptation: It is possible to improve safety and encourage independence by simplifying one's home to better suit the evolving demands of an Alzheimer's patient. This could entail eliminating risks, marking objects, creating schedules, and streamlining work to make it easier to handle.

Communication Techniques: Effective communication with people who have Alzheimer's disease can be facilitated by utilizing basic, uncomplicated communication tactics including speaking slowly, using visual cues, and asking yes/no questions. A great communication strategy also requires empathy, patience, and active listening.

Behavioral Management Strategies: Creating tailored strategies to address behavioral and psychological symptoms of Alzheimer's disease, like focusing attention in different directions, offering fulfilling activities, and maintaining a quiet and orderly environment, can help lessen agitation and enhance quality of life for both Alzheimer's patients and their carriers.

Caregivers' Self-Care: Caregivers' health and wellbeing depend on their making time for self-care and taking breaks from their caregiving responsibilities. This could be assigning responsibilities, establishing limits, taking part in stress-relieving activities, and asking friends, family, or trained caregivers for assistance.

A proactive, multimodal strategy that takes into account the special demands of both Alzheimer's patients and their carriers is needed to overcome the obstacles and challenges brought on by the disease.

Monitoring Progress and Adjusting Diet Accordingly

Monitoring Progress: Keeping tabs on the advance of Alzheimer's disease entails keeping an eye on alterations in mental abilities, conduct, and general health. Cognitive exams, behavioral assessments, and functional evaluations are just a few of the assessment instruments that caregivers and medical professionals can use to monitor changes over time. Frequent monitoring makes it possible to identify changes early and to take prompt action to successfully treat symptoms.

Key Dietary Strategies:

Stress the importance of eating a Mediterranean-style diet: this type of eating has been linked to a lower risk of Alzheimer's disease and cognitive decline. It is high in fruits, vegetables, whole grains, seafood, and olive oil. Promote a diet low in processed foods and refined sugars and high in plant-based foods, healthy fats, and lean proteins.

Boost your consumption of foods that help the brain: Include foods high in antioxidants (like berries, leafy greens, and nuts), omega-3 fatty acids (like salmon, walnuts, and flaxseeds), and vitamins (such vitamin B12 and E) in the diet. These nutrients may help slow down the onset of Alzheimer's disease and have been demonstrated to support brain health.

Keep yourself hydrated: Alzheimer's sufferers may experience worsening cognitive symptoms if they are dehydrated. Encourage drinking enough water, herbal teas, and fresh juices throughout the day. Keep a careful eye on the levels of hydration, particularly in people who might find it difficult to express their thirst.

Maximize nutrient absorption: Chewing, swallowing, and digestion issues might cause inadequate nutrient absorption in certain Alzheimer's patients. Serve nutrient-dense, easily chewed and digested foods, like purees, soups, and smoothies. If you require individualized meal planning or supplements, think about speaking with a nutritionist.

Adjusting Diet Accordingly: Dietary requirements and tastes may vary as Alzheimer's disease worsens. It's critical to maintain flexibility and modify the diet as necessary to accommodate each person's changing needs. Caregivers should monitor the effects of dietary modifications on symptoms and modify the diet as necessary. To preserve the person's autonomy and dignity, include them in the planning and preparation of meals.

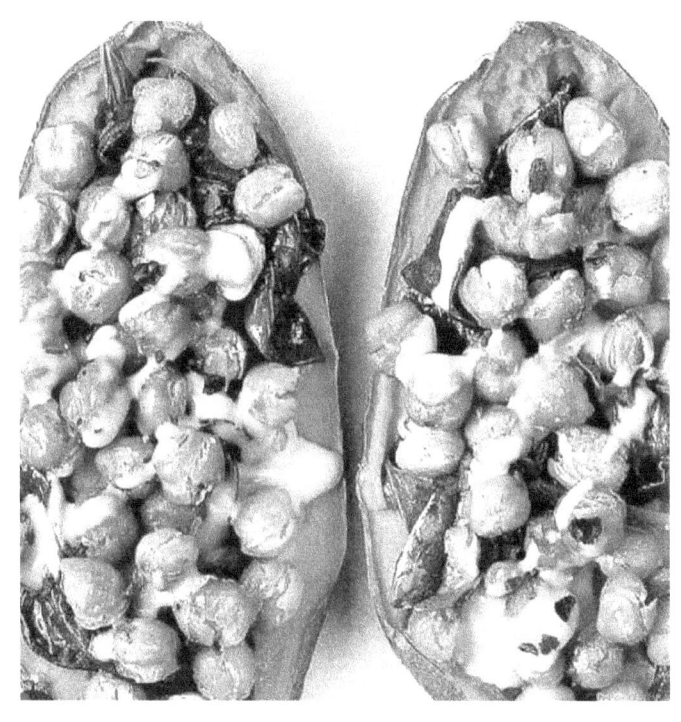

Practical Tips for Caregivers:

To monitor your nutritional consumption and spot trends or triggers, keep a food journal.
Provide regular, modest meals and snacks to keep energy levels up and hunger at bay.
Establish a stress-free, distraction-free dining space for your patrons.
Think about using supplements while being supervised by a medical practitioner.
Consult a qualified dietitian or nutritionist who specializes in Alzheimer's disease treatment for assistance.

One of the most important aspects of controlling Alzheimer's disease is keeping an eye on development and modifying the diet as needed. In order to enhance cognitive performance and general well-being in patients with Alzheimer's disease, caregivers should emphasize a healthy diet rich in nutrients that boost the brain and adjust to changing needs.

Through a comprehensive strategy that combines dietary interventions, medical care, and lifestyle changes, it is feasible to maintain dignity and improve quality of life even as the disease progresses.

It might be difficult to live with or care for someone who has Alzheimer's disease, but you are not alone. There are many of resources to help along the way with knowledge, encouragement, and support.

The resources provided in this guide can assist you in navigating the complexity of Alzheimer's disease and locating the support you require, whether you're looking for clinical trials, instructional materials, or caregiver support services. Recall that the best way to manage Alzheimer's disease and enhance the lives of both patients and caregivers is via education and support.

SEVEN (7) DAY MEDITERRENEAN MEAL PLAN FOR ALZHEIMERS DISEASE

A Mediterranean diet plan for Alzheimer's disease should include foods high in antioxidants, omega-3 fatty acids, vitamins, and minerals, and other nutrients that are good for the brain. Here is a seven-day meal plan specifically designed for those with Alzheimer's disease, based on the well-established cognitive benefits of the Mediterranean diet:

Day 1:
Breakfast: Consists of walnuts and Greek yogurt topped with berries (strawberries, raspberries, or blueberries).
Lunch: Grilled salmon salad dressed with cucumbers, cherry tomatoes, and mixed greens with a vinaigrette of olive oil.
Dinner: Quinoa topped with baked chicken breast and roasted veggies, like eggplant, zucchini, and bell peppers.

Day 2:
Breakfast: Consists of oatmeal with banana slices, almond slices, and honey drizzled on top.

Lunch: Consists of a whole grain wrap with grilled chicken, spinach, shredded carrots, and hummus inside.
Dinner: Whole grain bread-topped Mediterranean vegetable stew that includes chickpeas, tomatoes, spinach, and herbs.

Day 3:

Breakfast; Whole grain toast with spinach and feta omelet.
Lunch: Consists of a Greek salad (lettuce, tomatoes, cucumbers, olives, and feta cheese) and lentil soup.
Dinner: Lemon-dressed quinoa tabbouleh with grilled shrimp skewers and tomatoes, cucumbers, and parsley.

Day 4:

Breakfast: Almond milk, banana, Greek yogurt, spinach, and kale blended into a smoothie.
Lunch: Salad of whole grains and roasted veggies, like bell peppers, broccoli, and cherry tomatoes, dressed with balsamic vinegar and olive oil.
Dinner: Roasted potatoes, steamed green beans, and baked white fish, such as cod or tilapia.

Day 5:

Breakfast: Consists of avocado toast on whole grain bread with feta cheese and tomato slices on top.
Lunch: Quinoa salad topped with red onion, cherry tomatoes, sliced cucumber, chickpeas, and a lemon-herb vinaigrette.
Dinner: Roasted root vegetables (sweet potatoes, carrots,

and parsnips) paired with grilled lamb chops and tzatziki sauce.

Day 6:

Breakfast: Granola, honey, and mixed berries layered on top of a Greek yogurt parfait.
Lunch: A simple caprese salad dressed with olive oil and balsamic glaze, sliced tomatoes, and fresh mozzarella.
Dinner: Whole grain couscous with stuffed peppers prepared in the Mediterranean manner using ground turkey, quinoa, tomatoes, and herbs.

Day 7:

Breakfast: Consists of whole grain pancakes with mixed fruit compote (apples, peaches, or berries) and Greek yogurt on top.
Lunch: Consists of a whole grain pita filled with lettuce, tomato, cucumber, falafel, and tahini sauce.
Dinner: Wild rice on the side, roasted asparagus, and baked fish in a lemon-dill sauce.

As you work through the day, don't forget to stay hydrated by consuming lots of water and adding nutritious snacks like nuts, seeds, and fresh fruit as needed. The focus of this meal plan is on complete, nutrient-dense foods that promote general health and brain function.

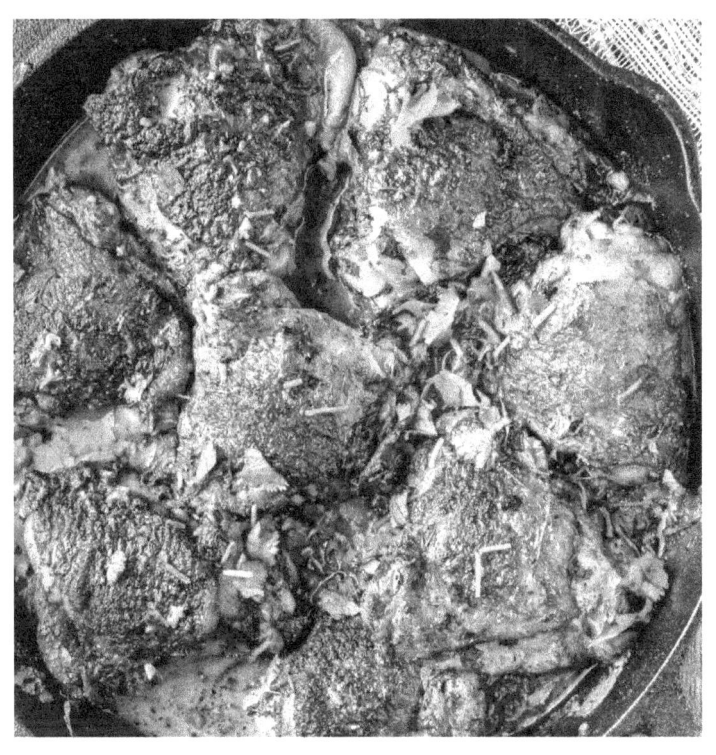

CONCLUSION

In the struggle against cognitive loss, "Mediterranean Diet for Alzheimer's Disease" is a ray of empowerment and hope. Readers have traveled on a voyage of discovery via the pages of this life-changing book, discovering the fundamental relationship between nutrition and mental health.

The Mediterranean diet has become a powerful tool in maintaining cognitive function and preventing Alzheimer's disease because of its availability of healthful foods like fruits, vegetables, whole grains, fish, and olive oil.

It's clear from our examination of the plethora of enlightening tales and scientific studies that following a Mediterranean diet isn't only about feeding the body; it's also about feeding the mind. The testimonials included in these chapters attest to the miraculous effects of minor dietary adjustments, giving Alzheimer's patients and their loved one's newfound hope.

This book is more than just a collection of dietary guidelines; it's a call to action, a reminder that every meal presents an opportunity to improve brain function. When we follow the guidelines of the Mediterranean diet, we not only strengthen our brains but also add flavor and nutritious food to our life.

May this book be your road map to the best possible brain health, giving you the knowledge and skills to make decisions that promote cognitive vibrancy and improve general wellbeing. Together, with knowledge, resiliency, and a dedication to preserving humankind's most valuable resource—the brain—let's set off on this journey.

BONUS EXERCISE PROGRAM FOR ALZHEIMERS DISEASE

EXERCISE FOR YOUR BRAIN

Crosswords

Dance

Jigsaw puzzles

Learning

Sudoku

Vocabulary

Listening to music

Reading

Socialize

Card games

There's no denying that regular exercise promotes better health. It helps to manage weight, drop blood pressure, raise blood sugar, reduce waist circumference, increase fitness, elevate mood, and lessen anxiety. These advantages are particularly crucial for Alzheimer's patients, who frequently experience mood swings and co-occurring chronic illnesses.

Additionally, regular exercise can help people with Alzheimer's disease slow down their condition's progressive cognitive loss. Alzheimer's patients and their caregivers may be unsure about what kinds of activities are safe to perform on a regular basis. What form of exercise, then, is recommended for those who have Alzheimer's disease?

A simple method for considering suitable exercise for those with Alzheimer's disease is the FITT model. The terms "frequency, intensity, time, and type of exercise" are referred to as FITT. For those suffering from Alzheimer's disease, the US government has provided guidelines for exercise that encompass every aspect of the FITT model.

People with Alzheimer's disease may benefit from exercise because it can help maintain physical function, boost mood, and possibly slow down cognitive decline. But before beginning any new fitness routine, it's critical to speak with a healthcare provider and customize the program to the person's skills and preferences.

The following general guidelines can be used to create a fitness program for an individual who has Alzheimer's disease:

1. Assessment: Prior to beginning any fitness regimen, it is critical to evaluate the person's present level of physical fitness, health history, and potential dangers. A medical

practitioner, such as a doctor or physical therapist, can perform this assessment.

2.Exercise Types: Include a range of workouts that target many facets of fitness, such as:

Aerobic Exercise: Exercises like walking, swimming, cycling, or dancing that raise heart rate and respiration are referred to as aerobic exercises. Aim for 150 minutes or more a week of moderate-to-intense aerobic activity, or as tolerated.

Strength Training: Involves the use of resistance bands, light weights, or bodyweight movements like squats and modified push-ups to target the primary muscle groups. Incorporate strength training activities two to three times a week, emphasizing safety and good form.

Balancing and Coordination: Practices like yoga, tai chi, or particular balancing exercises suggested by a physical therapist that enhance balance and coordination. Fall risk can be decreased with the aid of these activities.

Flexibility and Stretching: Yoga and Pilates are two gentle stretching workouts that help increase range of motion and flexibility. It's important to stretch frequently, ideally every day, to keep your body flexible and avoid becoming stiff.

3.Safety Measures:
Always put safety first and begin with workouts suitable for the person's present fitness level and capabilities. Make sure the workout area is safe and devoid of risks that could lead to falls or injuries, and utilize the appropriate equipment.

When exercising, keep an eye out for any signs of exhaustion, pain, or overexertion and modify the time or intensity as necessary.
Drink plenty of water and take breaks when needed, particularly in warm or muggy conditions.

4. Consistency and Adaptation:
Create a regular workout schedule and try to fit in physical activity whenever you can.
Be ready to modify the exercise regimen as needed to accommodate a person's evolving needs, preferences, or state of health.

5. Supervision and Assistance:
Offer guidance and assistance to the person exercising, particularly if they have cognitive limitations or safety concerns.

To promote motivation and social contact, encourage participation in group exercise programs or activities.

6. Pleasure and Involvement:
Select pursuits that the person finds fulfilling and pleasurable, since this can boost drive and commitment to the fitness regimen.
To add some fun and cerebral stimulation to your workout, mix in entertaining activities like games or music.

Keep in mind that each person with Alzheimer's disease is different, so it's critical to tailor the exercise regimen to their particular requirements, capabilities, and preferences. It is possible to maintain the safety, efficacy, and enjoyment of the exercise program by maintaining regular communication with medical experts, caregivers, and family members.